FIRST AID
for Nurses

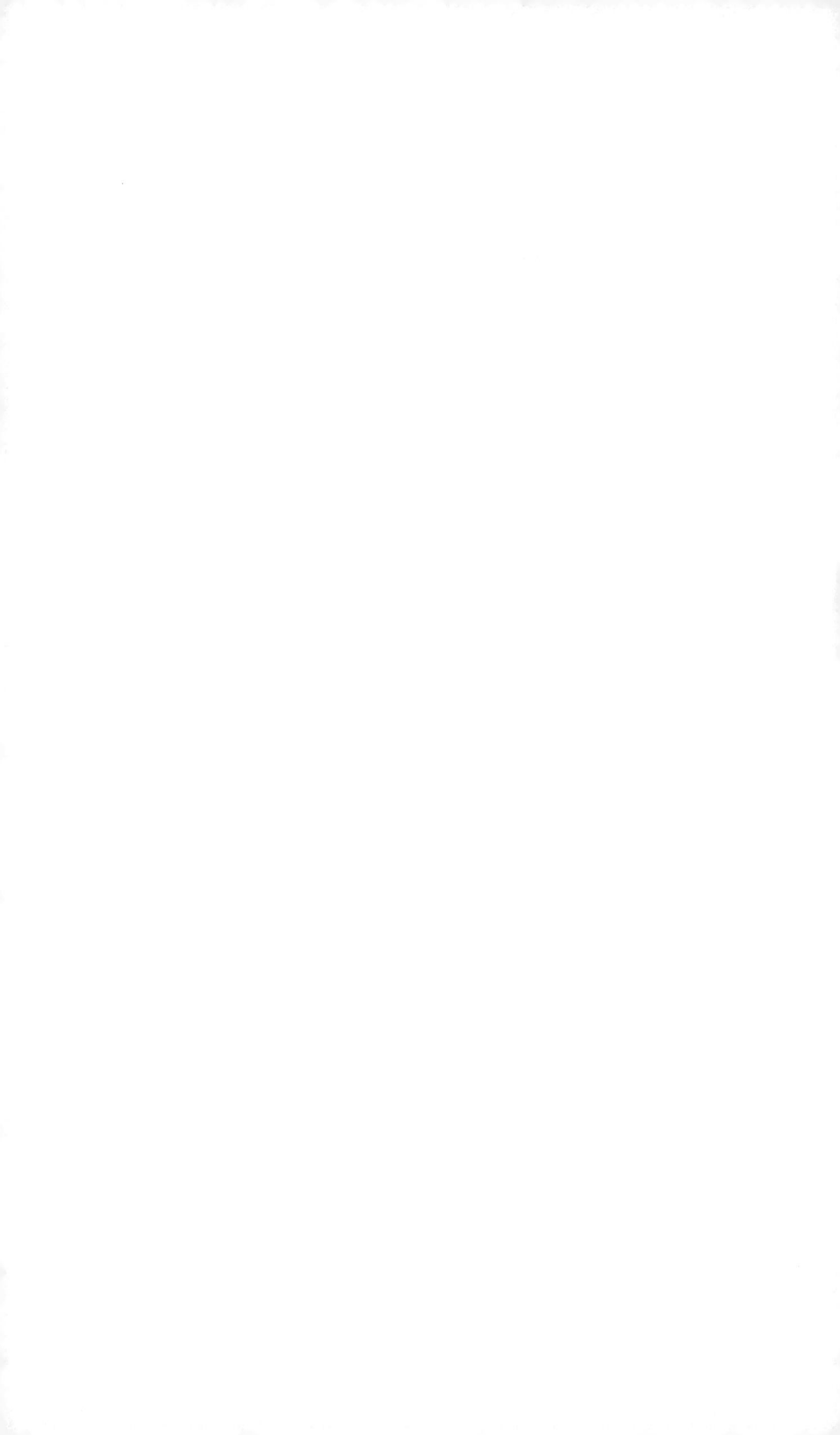

FIRST AID
for Nurses

(As per the Nursing Syllabus)

Third Edition

TK Indrani BSc (N)
Ex-Assistant Lecturer
College of Nursing
Sri Ramachandra Medical College and
Research Institute (Deemed University)
Chennai, Tamil Nadu, India

Teresa Lamniang
MSN Mental Health (Psychiatry) Nursing
RNRM BSc (H) Nursing
New Delhi, India

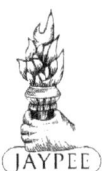

JAYPEE BROTHERS MEDICAL PUBLISHERS
The Health Sciences Publisher
New Delhi | London

Jaypee Brothers Medical Publishers (P) Ltd

Headquarters
Jaypee Brothers Medical Publishers (P) Ltd
EMCA House, 23/23-B
Ansari Road, Daryaganj
New Delhi 110 002, India
Landline: +91-11-23272143, +91-11-23272703
+91-11-23282021, +91-11-23245672
Email: jaypee@jaypeebrothers.com

Overseas Office
J.P. Medical Ltd
83 Victoria Street, London
SW1H 0HW (UK)
Phone: +44 20 3170 8910
Email: info@jpmedpub.com

Corporate Office
Jaypee Brothers Medical Publishers (P) Ltd
4838/24, Ansari Road, Daryaganj
New Delhi 110 002, India
Phone: +91-11-43574357
Fax: +91-11-43574314
Email: jaypee@jaypeebrothers.com

EU GPSR Authorised Representative
Logos Europe, 9 rue Nicolas Poussin
17000, La Rochelle, France
Phone: +33 (0) 6 67 93 73 78
E-mail: Contact@logoseurope.eu

Website: www.jaypeebrothers.com
Website: www.jaypeedigital.com

© 2024, Jaypee Brothers Medical Publishers

The views and opinions expressed in this book are solely those of the original contributor(s)/author(s) and do not necessarily represent those of editor(s) and publisher of the book.

All rights reserved. No part of this publication may be reproduced, stored or transmitted in any form or by any means, electronic, mechanical, photocopying, recording or otherwise, without the prior permission in writing of the publishers.

All brand names and product names used in this book are trade names, service marks, trademarks or registered trademarks of their respective owners. The publisher is not associated with any product or vendor mentioned in this book.

Medical knowledge and practice change constantly. This book is designed to provide accurate, authoritative information about the subject matter in question. However, readers are advised to check the most current information available on procedures included and check information from the manufacturer of each product to be administered, to verify the recommended dose, formula, method and duration of administration, adverse effects and contraindications. It is the responsibility of the practitioner to take all appropriate safety precautions. Neither the publisher nor the author(s)/editor(s) assume any liability for any injury and/or damage to persons or property arising from or related to use of material in this book.

This book is sold on the understanding that the publisher is not engaged in providing professional medical services. If such advice or services are required, the services of a competent medical professional should be sought.

Every effort has been made where necessary to contact holders of copyright to obtain permission to reproduce copyright material. If any have been inadvertently overlooked, the publisher will be pleased to make the necessary arrangements at the first opportunity.

Inquiries for bulk sales may be solicited at: jaypee@jaypeebrothers.com

First Aid for Nurses

First Edition: 2003

Reprint 2005, 2006, 2008

Second Edition: 2018

Third Edition: **2024**

ISBN: 978-93-5696-365-8

Dedicated to

*Jaypee Brothers Medical Publishers (P) Ltd
for
showing keen interest to publish this book*

Preface to the Third Edition

In the healthcare profession, nurses are the compassionate healers, advocates, and undertake relentless pursuit of knowledge. Nurses are resilient and with an unwavering commitment to those in need, they have a crucial role in the frontline of emergencies, both in hospital settings and in the broader community. With this immense pride and dedication we present the third edition of *First Aid for Nurses* curated with the unique needs of life-saving knowledge for nurses in mind. In this book, we embark on an updated knowledge of first aid, where prompt and skilled responses can often be the difference between life and loss.

Our goal with this book is to provide a resource that empowers nurses, other healthcare professionals as well as the general public to deliver prompt and proficient first aid in emergency situations. The information contained in this book is designed and curated based on the latest updated first aid module and according to the revised INC syllabus. In these chapters, we delve into the fundamentals of first aid from the assessment to the application of life-saving techniques and including the art of decision-making in emergencies. These topics are analyzed in the book comprehensively in an easy to understand method.

We hope the third edition will be of great use for nursing students, faculty and all nurses who stand ready to offer comfort in the moment of crisis and emergency situations.

TK Indrani
Teresa Lamniang

Preface to the First Edition

First aid and medical aid are two interrelated concepts which are used to provide immediate and on-the-spot treatment to the victim of an accident or sudden illness. As lifestyles of people are becoming more complex and changing rapidly affecting various aspects of their living environment, it is imperative that every person should be capable of rendering first aid to sick and injured person till the patient reaches in the safe hands of specific medical personnel.

Although *First Aid for Nurses* is intended primarily to provide sufficient knowledge to medical fellows particularly nursing professionals, a common man can emerge as skilled first aider when he follows the guidelines of the book strictly. It provides sufficient coverage of all critical situations resulting from accidental or sudden illness of patients which require primarily first aid, instead of a complex medical assistance, to save the life of the patient. Asphyxia, resuscitation, shocks, excessive hemorrhage, fractures, burns, poisoning, etc. are such critical situations which need to be handled with great dexterity by the first aider. These topics are analyzed in the book comprehensively in an easy to understand method. Community emergency is a broad concept which deals not only with an individual situation, but also the people at large. So, a macro view is attempted in handling first aid in community emergency. It also describes in great detail the bandaging procedures and dressing materials received by the first aider. In this connection, a First Aid Atlas is being given in the book which provides figures on different aspects of critical cases and bandaging procedures.

I hope the book will bring positive response from readers whose comments and remarks are welcome for further improvement of the book.

TK Indrani

Acknowledgments

"Gratitude is the fairest blossom that springs from the soul."
—**Henry Ward Beecher**
This quote beautifully encapsulates the sentiment of acknowledge and gratitude. The creation of *First Aid for Nurses* has been a collaborative effort that would not have been possible without the support, expertize, and dedication of many individuals and organization. We would like to express our heartfelt gratitude to all those who have contributed to the realization of this book.

First and foremost, we extend our deepest appreciation to the nurses who are the heart and soul of this book. Your unwavering commitment to patient care, your tireless dedication to learning, and your invaluable insights have shaped every aspect of this work.

We are extremely grateful to Shri Jitendar P Vij (Group Chairman), Mr Ankit Vij (Managing Director) and Mr MS Mani (Group President) who are the continual source of inspiration throughout this journey.

We are immensely grateful to Dr Madhu Choudhary (Director-Educational Publishing) for her guidance, mentorship and support in enriching the content of this book.

A special note of thanks goes to my colleagues Ms Alisha, Ms Jitika, Dr Aditya and Dr Sneha who shared their expertize and insights during the creation of this book. Their encouragement and motivation has been a driving force.

We express our sincere gratitude and appreciation to the team of Jaypee Brothers Medical Publishers (P) Ltd, New Delhi, India, especially Ms Pooja Bhandari [Director-Production (Books and Journals)], Ms Sunita Katla (Executive Assistant to Group Chairman and Publishing Manager), Ms Samina Khan (Executive assistant to Director-Educational Publishing) and Mr Rajesh Sharma (Production Coordinator) for their constant efforts and support throughout this project.

We extend our gratitude to Ms Seema Dogra (Cover Visualizer), Ms Neelam Kakriya (Proof Reader), Mr Kulwant Singh (Typesetter) and Rakesh Verma (Graphic Designer), their dedication, expertize

Acknowledgements

and attention to details have been instrumental in making this project a reality.

Our deepest gratitude goes to our families, whose support and understanding have been a valuable encouragement throughout the process of creating this book.

We express our heartfelt thanks to the readers of this book. It is our sincere hope that the knowledge and insights contained within these pages will enhance your understanding of first aid in nursing and contribute to the betterment of patient care.

Contents

SECTION 1: INTRODUCTION TO FIRST AID

Chapter 1: First Aid   3
- Definition   3
- Outline of First Aid   3
- Scope of First Aid   4
- Management of Case   5
- Golden Rules of First Aid   6
- Action at an Emergency (Concept of Emergency)   7

Chapter 2: Essential Body Parts: Structure and Functions   20
- Musculoskeletal System   22
- Respiratory System   26
- Digestive System   27
- Circulatory System   28
- Endocrine System   29
- Sensory Organs   30
- Excretory System   31
- Reproductive System   31
- Nervous System   32
- Integumentary System   33

SECTION 2: FIRST AID MANAGEMENT

Chapter 3: Wounds, Hemorrhage and Shock   37

3.1: Wounds   37
- Definition   38
- Types of Wound   38

3.2: Hemorrhage   53
- Definition   53
- Classification   53
- Common Signs and Symptoms of Hemorrhage   54
- First Aid Measures of Hemorrhage/Bleeding   54

3.3: Shock   68
- Definition   68

- Causes 68
- Stages of Shock 69
- Classification of Shock 69
- Signs and Symptoms 70
- First Aid Management 71

Chapter 4: Musculoskeletal Injuries 73

4.1: Fracture, Muscle Injuries and Dislocation 73
- Fracture 73
- First Aid Injuries to Joints and Muscles 80

4.2: Injuries: Head, Spinal Cord and Others 85
- Head Injuries 85
- Spinal Injury 87
- Others 89

4.3: Bandages and Dressings 93
- Bandages 93

Chapter 5: Transportation of Injured Persons 114
- Transport of Injured Persons 114
- Methods of Transportation 114

Chapter 6: Respiratory Emergencies and Basic CPR 128

6.1: Respiratory Emergencies 128
- Asphyxia 128
- Choking 131
- External Obstruction 134
- Suffocation 134
- Asthma 136
- Smoke Inhalation 137
- Drowning 137
- Hanging, Strangling and Throttling 139

6.2: Emergency Resuscitation 141
- Victim Assessment 141
- Airway Obstruction 143
- Basic Life Support (Resuscitation) 145

Chapter 7: Unconsciousness 154
- Common Causes of Unconsciousness 155

Chapter 8: Foreign Bodies 166
- Splinters 166
- Foreign Body in the Eye 167
- Foreign Body in the Ear 168
- Foreign Body in the Nose 169
- Foreign Body in the Throat 170
- Foreign Body in the Stomach 170

Chapter 9: Burns and Scalds — 171
- Definition *171*
- Burns *172*

Chapter 10: Poisoning, Bites and Stings — 187

10.1: Poisoning 187
- Definition of Poison *187*
- Mode of Poison Entry Into the Body *187*
- Poison Action and Effects *188*
- Poisoning Determination by First Aider *189*
- General Rules For the Treatment of Poisoning *191*
- Types of Poisons *193*
- Sources of Various Poisons, Clinical Features and First Aid Measures *206*

10.2: Bites and Stings 209
- Insects *209*
- Spiders *210*
- Snakes *213*
- Scorpion Sting *219*
- Bee, Wasp and Hornet Stings *219*
- Jellyfish Sting *220*
- Portuguese Man-of-War *220*
- Sea Urchin Sting *220*
- Cone-shaped Shells *221*
- Coral Cuts *221*
- Rabies and Antirabic Treatment in India *221*

Chapter 11: Frostbite and Effects of Heat — 225
- Frostbite *225*
- Effects of Heat/Extreme Temperature *227*

Chapter 12: Community Emergencies — 232

12.1: Disaster Management 232
- Definitions *233*
- Types of Disasters *233*
- Causes of Disaster *234*
- Effects of Disaster *237*
- Management Disaster *238*
- Disaster Management *239*

12.2: First Aid Kit 260
- Contents of First Aid Kit *260*
- Injuries and First Aid Supplies to be used *262*

Index 263

Syllabus

FIRST AID

*Syllabus for First aid is given in Unit XIV of Nursing Foundation-I
Placement: I Semester
Theory (T): 20 Hours
Skill Lab (SL): 20 Hours

Unit	Time (Hrs)	Learning Outcomes	Content	Teaching/ Learning Activities	Assessment Methods

XIV	20 (T) 20 (SL)	Explain and apply principles of First Aid during emergencies	**First Aid***
			 • Definition, Basic Principles, Scope and Rules
			 • First Aid Management:
			   o Wounds, Hemorrhage and Shock
			   o Musculoskeletal Injuries—Fractures, Dislocation, Muscle injuries
			   o Transportation of Injured persons
			   o Respiratory Emergencies and Basic CPR
			   o Unconsciousness
			   o Foreign Bodies—Skin, Eye, Ear, Nose, Throat and Stomach
			   o Burns and Scalds
			   o Poisoning, Bites and Stings
			   o Frostbite and Effects of Heat
			   o Community Emergencies
				• Lecture
				 • Discussion
				 • Demonstration and Re-demonstration
				 • Module completion
				 • National Disaster Management Authority (NDMA)/ Indian Red Cross Society (IRCS) and First Aid module
					• Essay
					 • Short answer
					 • Objective type
					 • OSCE

Introduction to First Aid

Chapter 1: First Aid

Chapter 2: Essential Body Parts: Structure and Functions

First Aid

CHAPTER 1

CHAPTER OUTLINE

- Scope of First Aid
- First Aider Management of Case
- Golden Rules of First Aid
- Action at an Emergency
- C-A-B
- Calling for Assistance
- How to Carry Out Examination
- Levels of Responsiveness

INTRODUCTION

The term 'first aid' was adopted officially in England for the first time in 1879 by the St John Ambulance Association. The expression 'first aid' had not come till 1894 and intended to designate any person who has received a certificate from an authorized association that he/she is qualified to render first aid.

DEFINITION

First aid is the immediate and temporary care given to the victim of an accident or sudden illness. Its purpose is to preserve life, assist recovery and prevent aggravation of the condition until the services of a doctor can be obtained or during transportation to hospital or to the casualty's home.

OUTLINE OF FIRST AID

The principles and practice of first aid are based on the principles of practical medicine and surgery, knowledge of which, in case of accident or sudden illness, enables trained persons to give such skilled assistance that will preserve life, promote recovery and prevent the injury or illness becoming worse until medical aid has been obtained.

The term 'medical aid' is used to indicate treatment by a doctor either on the spot, in the home or in hospital. The first aider's responsibilities ends as soon as medical aid is available, but he/she should standby after making his/her report to the doctor in case he/she can be of further assistance.

First aid is definitely limited to the assistance rendered at the time of emergency with whatever resources that may be available. It is not intended that the first aider should take the place of the doctor or medical professionals, and it must be clearly understood that the redressing of injuries and other such after treatment are outside the scope of first aid.

Throughout the manual, standard methods of treatment are given for a number of defined conditions, which may occur in different circumstances, but the first aider will find that these conditions seldom conform to an exact pattern and that even in the same circumstances individuals may react in different ways. He/she must be prepared to sum up any situation with which he/she may be faced and adapt himself/herself to wide variation from the average or typical.

SCOPE OF FIRST AID

- ❖ **Diagnosis:** To determine the nature of the case requiring attention for the purpose of intelligent and efficient treatment.
- ❖ **Treatment:** To determine the nature and extent of the treatment until medical aid is available.
- ❖ **Disposal:** Transport the casualty to the nearest shelter, either to his/her home or clinic or hospital.

Diagnosis

In deciding nature of the case, first aider must consider the following:
- ❖ History
- ❖ Symptoms
- ❖ Signs

History

History is the story of how an accident or sudden illness occurred. This may be obtained from the casualty (if conscious) or from witnesses. It may be information that a person is subject to a particular disease or the surroundings may suggest the cause, e.g., a broken bicycle.

Symptoms

Symptoms are the sensations of the casualty such as feeling cold or shivery, faintness, nausea, thirst pain, which can be obtained, if conscious casualty describes. Pain is a very helpful diagnostic point for the first aider as it draws his/her attention to the part, which is most probably in trouble and saves a great deal of time during his/her examination of the casualty.

Signs

Signs are any variations from the normal conditions of the casualty such as pallor, congestion, swelling and deformity, which can be observed by the first aider. Signs are the most reliable indications on which to base diagnosis, but the circumstances of each particular case will determine the relative importance of history, symptoms and signs.

Treatment

If the cause of the condition is still active, remove the cause if possible (e.g., a log of wood on leg), or remove the casualty from the cause of the conditions (e.g., gas-filled room). Give treatment to preserve life, promote recovery and prevent the condition becoming worse. Pay special attention to the treatment of failure of breathing, severe bleeding and shock. When there is the slightest doubt as to whether a casualty is dead or alive, continue treatment until medical aid has been obtained.

Disposal

The speed with which a casualty is brought under medical care is of tremendous importance in his/her recovery. Unless the casualty is examined by a doctor on the spot, it is the responsibility of the first aider to see that he/she is conveyed to his/her home (or other suitable temporary shelter) or to hospital as soon as possible in the manner most suitable in the circumstances. A tactful message should be sent to the casualty's home or relatives indicating in a general way, 'what has happened and the casualty's destination'.

MANAGEMENT OF CASE

The first aider must always:
- Respond quickly to calls for assistance, the saving of a life may depend on promptness of action.
- Adopt a calm and methodical approach to the casualty, quick and confident examination, and treatment, which will relieve pain and distress, lessen the effect of the injury and may save life. Time spent

on long and elaborate examination of a casualty may be time lost in his/her ultimate recovery.
- ❖ Treat obvious injuries and conditions endangering life such as failure of breathing and severe shock, before making a complete diagnosis.
- ❖ Take first aid material, if this is immediately available. If standard equipment is not available, the first aider must depend on material at hand, which will have to be improvise as required.
- ❖ Study the surroundings carefully. These may influence the action to be taken and therefore require careful consideration, for example:

> - **Danger:** From falling building, moving machinery, electric current, fire, poisonous gases and similar hazards.
> - **Weather:** If the accident occurs out-of-doors, the casualty may be treated in the open air if the weather is fine; if the weather is bad, he/she must be removed to shelter as soon as is reasonably possible.
> - **Shelter:** Houses and buildings near at hand, whether occupied or unoccupied, and whether likely to be particularly useful (e.g., a chemist's shop), otherwise, temporary shelter may be provided by means of umbrellas, rugs, etc.
> - **Light:** It is impossible to treat a patient satisfactorily without sufficient light, and the first aider must provide for this.
> - **Assistance:** Crowds must be tactfully controlled. If a doctor is present, work under his/her direction. If not, ask if anyone with knowledge of first aid is present. If neither is available make use of bystanders to the best advantage.
> - **Reassure the casualty:** By speaking encouragingly, warn him/her to be still and tell that he/she is in trained hands.

GOLDEN RULES OF FIRST AID

- ❖ Do "first thing first": Assessing the situation for immediate danger, quickly and methodically without panicking, give first priority to urgent condition.
- ❖ Remove the victim from the cause of injury or the cause of injury from the victim (do not move a victim unless you really have to)
- ❖ Resuscitate the victim, if necessary.
- ❖ Carry out general treatment of unconsciousness (in case of unconscious victim).
- ❖ Loosen all tight clothing or materials around the victim's neck waist, wrist, etc.

- Stop bleeding, cover all wounds, burns or scalds and immobilize all fractures.
- Separate victim from crowd.
- Reassure the victim and get help as soon as possible.
- If materials are not available, improvise.
- Guide against or treat for shock.
- Transport the victim properly.

ACTION AT AN EMERGENCY (CONCEPT OF EMERGENCY)

The basic principles of first aid apply to all injuries or illnesses regardless of severity. Whatever the incident, it is the first aider's responsibility to act quickly, calmly and correctly in order to:
- Preserve life
- Prevent deterioration in the casualty's condition
- Promote recovery.

These objectives are best achieved by:
- A rapid, but calm approach
- A quick assessment of the situation and the casualty
- A correct diagnosis of the condition based on the history of the incident and the casualty's history, symptoms and signs
- Immediate and appropriate treatment of any conditions diagnosed
- Proper disposal of the casualty according to the injury or condition.

> **THE FIRST ACTIONS BY FIRST AIDERS: DR CAB**
> **D** – Danger assessment for self and victim
> **R** – Responsiveness of the victim
> **C** – Check and assess for pulse
> **A** – Assess and ensure clear airway
> **B** – Check if person is breathing

Approach

Approach should be speedy, but calm and controlled. Ensure that you are not placing yourself in any danger when approaching the casualty. On arrival at the scene of any incident, state that you are a trained first aider and, if there are no doctors, nurses or more experienced people present, calmly take charge.

General Rules

Whenever and wherever you come across an emergency, use common sense, know the limitations and do not attempt to do too much.

Assessing the Situation

As soon as you have taken control at an incident, it is crucial to make an accurate assessment of the situation and decide on the priorities of action. To do this you must consider:
- Whether you and the casualty are not in any danger
- If the casualty has any life-threatening conditions
- If any bystanders can help you
- Whether you need to call for assistance

Safety

You must minimize the risk of danger to yourself, the casualty and bystanders, and guard against any further casualties arising (for example, in the case of road accidents).

Road Accidents

Instruct a bystander to control traffic, keeping it well away from yourself and the casualty. Watch out for life risks, especially from petrol spillage and switch off the ignition of the vehicles concerned.

Determining Priorities

- In order to determine the condition of a casualty, ask him/her "what happened?"
- A reply will help you to know what to look for
- It also tells you that he/she is conscious; his/her airway is clear; he/she is able to breathe, if he/she does not respond to questioning or touch, perform the following checks immediately.

Circulation/Chest Compression, Airway, Breathing (C-A-B)

- **Circulation:** Absence of breathing means patient's heart has stopped. Chest compression must be initiated to pump blood, particularly to the brain. This will help in restoring blood circulation.
- **Airway:** In case of unresponsive patient, tongue may block the airway. Manage by giving artificial ventilation **(Figs. 1.1A and B)**. These actions draw the tongue forward away from the back of the throat.

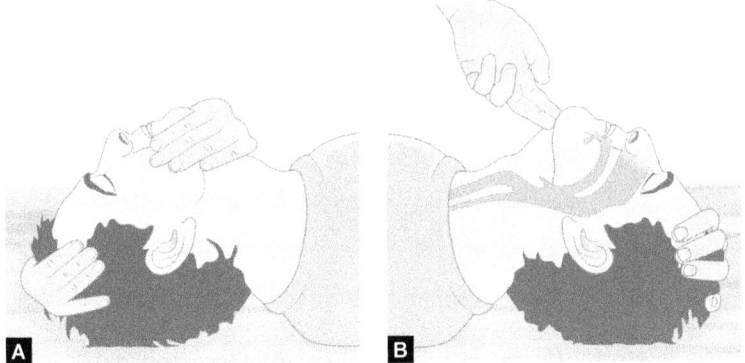

Figs. 1.1A and B: Artificial respiration: (A) Head-tilt, chin-lift; (B) Patency of airway.

- **Breathing:** Look, listen and feel for breathing. If patient is not breathing, then mouth-to-mouth resuscitation should be initiated.

> **Patient assessment is change from A-B-C to C-A-B method for the following reason:**
> - Chest compressions and early defibrillation are helpful in the management of pulseless ventricular tachycardia (VT).
> - Initial airway management delayed the initiation of chest compression.
> - Initial chest compression management will increase important bystander intervention, as significant obstacle to bystanders performing CPR is their fear of doing mouth-to-mouth breathing.

Unconsciousness

Place an unconscious casualty in the recover position as shown in **Figure 1.2** and assess the level of responsiveness.

If there is any possibility of spinal injury, do not turn the casualty and keep in spinal recovery position (refer topic 'examining the spine') unless difficulty in breathing makes it essential, or vomiting is likely to occur:

- **Gas and poisonous fumes:** If possible cut off the source and ensure adequate ventilation.
- **Electrical contact:** Break the contact, if possible, and take the necessary precautions against further contact.
- **Fire and collapsing buildings:** Move the casualty to safety immediately, if you can do so without endangering your own life.

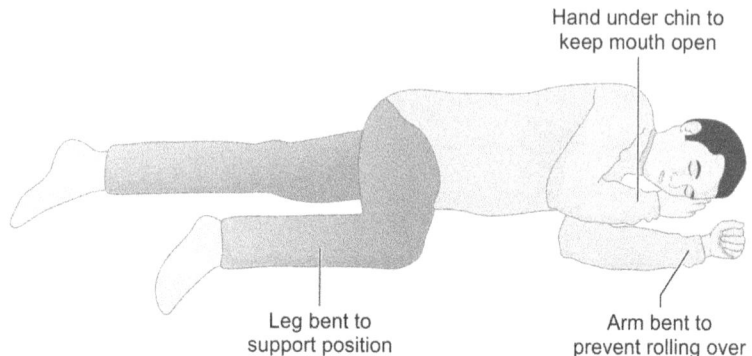

Fig. 1.2: Unconscious patient placed in recovery position.

Getting Others to Help You

Some bystanders can be extremely useful and may be able to assist with treatment. For example:
- Controlling severe bleeding or supporting a badly injured limb.
- Keep other bystanders occupied by asking them to control traffic, crowd or call for help.
- When asking bystander to make a phone call for help, make sure that they understand the message that is to be sent (ask them to write it down or make them repeat the message to you).
- Always make sure that bystanders report back to you after they are done with the phone call.

Shock

Keep the casualty warm, quiet and lying down until skilled help arrives. Refer Chapter 3.3 for detailed discussion of shock and its first aid management.

Other Needs

Unless there is immediate danger to life from the surroundings, treat all fractures and large wounds before moving a casualty. If the casualty is in danger, support the injured part whilst moving or if you suspect that the casualty has a fractured spine.

Calling for Assistance

Once you decide that assistance is required, and this may include ambulance, police, fire brigade, gas or electricity boards, send for it immediately. Call for the ambulance service required.

Do not leave the casualty unattended. Whether you are giving the message yourself or instructing someone to do so make sure that the following information is passed on:
1. Your telephone number.
2. The exact location of the incident; if you can point out nearby road junctions for other landmarks.
3. An indication of the type and seriousness of the incident, e.g., road traffic accident, two cars involved, three people trapped.
4. The number, sex and approximate age of the casualties involved and if possible, the nature of their injuries.
5. Request for special help and if you suspect a heart attack or childbirth.

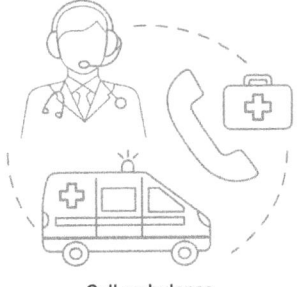
Call ambulance

Multiple Casualties and Injuries

Where there is more than one casualty, you must decide by rapid assessment, which one needs priority of treatment. Remember that the noisiest casualty is rarely the most severely injured. In first aid, common sense is almost as important as the actual knowledge of the subject.

In real life, serious accidents rarely produce only a single injury, frequently two or more injuries occur so that the correct treatment of one may interfere with the correct treatment of the other. In such circumstances you must decide, which injury is the more serious one and treat that in the correct way. You should then deal with the other injuries correctly as possible under the conflicting circumstances.

Examination and Diagnosis

Examination and diagnosis means taking account of the casualty's history and that of the incident, the symptoms, signs and levels of responsiveness.

How to Carry Out an Examination?

A general examination should be carried out quickly to discern any imminent threats to life whether the casualty is conscious or unconscious when examining a casualty. There are certain rules to follow:

- Move him/her as little as possible to avoid aggravating any injuries.
- Begin examination at the head and work methodically towards his/her feet.
- Remember to use all your senses—look, feel, listen and smell.
- Always compare one side of the casualty's body with the other as this makes it easier to detect any swellings or irregularities that require first aid.

> **Note:**
> If at any stage during the examination, the casualty's breathing becomes noisy and difficult, place the casualty in the recovery position.

Physical Examination

Examining the head

Mouth

Recheck breathing, noting the rate, depth and nature (whether easy or difficult, noisy or quiet); note also any odor. Check inside of the mouth to ensure it contains no foreign matter, such as vomit, blood, food or loose teeth that might cause choking.

Lips

Examine the lips for any signs of burning or discoloration that might indicate corrosive poisoning. Look inside the lips for blueness, which might indicate asphyxia.

Teeth

Check the teeth to make sure that any recently dislodged teeth have not fallen down into the back of the throat. Make sure that dentures are firm fitting (essential for resuscitation); if they are not, remove them.

Eyes

Examine both together comparing the pupils (the black circular centers) and noting whether they are equal in size. Check the white orbit of the eye for bloodshot.

Nose

Check for signs of blood, clear fluid or a mixture of both, which might come from inside the skull.

Face

Look at the color—it may be pale, flushed or even bluish if breathing is affected. At the same time, feel the temperature of the face to check whether it is particularly hot or cold and note the state of the skin whether it is dry or clammy or even sweating profusely.

Ears
Check the ears for foreign bodies and traces of blood and/or clear cerebrospinal fluid that might indicate skull fracture. Speak into the casualty's ears to test hearing.

Skull
Gently run the hands over the scalp searching for bleeding, swelling or any indentation that might indicate a fracture.

Examining the spine
- Loosen clothing around the neck.
- Run your fingers over the spine from the base of the skull down to as far as you can reach between the shoulders, checking for any irregularity of the vertebrae that might indicate a fracture.
- Check round the neck, to see whether any warning medallion is being worn.
- Check the carotid pulse **(Fig. 1.3)**, and note its rate, strength and rhythm.
- Note the presence or absence of movement or feeling in the casualty's limbs.

Examining the trunk
- Check the chest for evenness of rib movement or breathing and note any wounds that are 'sucking air.'

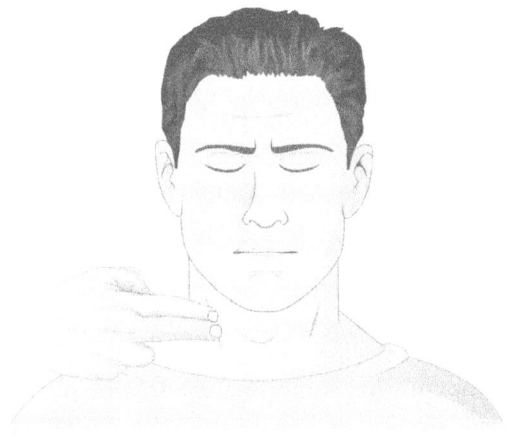

Fig. 1.3: Carotid pulse checking.

- Check the ribs for irregularity or depression that might indicate a fracture and also feel along the line of the breast bone.
- Check both collarbones for irregularity and the shoulders for signs of deformity. Carefully feel either side of the pelvis looking for signs of fracture and note any indication of incontinence.

Examining the arms

Examine the upper arm bones, then the bones in the forearm, wrists, hands and fingers. Check carefully for any deformity and swelling, which might indicate fractures. Check the forearms to see if the casualty is wearing a medical warning bracelet and for injection marks. Needle marks might indicate either drug abuse or diabetes.

Examining the legs

Check the hips, thighs, knee caps, both bones of the lower legs, the ankles, feet and toes in the same way as the arms.

> **Note:**
> Use two hands so that you can examine and compare both sides of the body at the same time.

Levels of Responsiveness

There are various stages through which a casualty may pass during progression from consciousness to unconsciousness. If the casualty responds well to stimulation then unconsciousness is only light (e.g., as in a faint). However, he/she is still in a potentially dangerous state. If the response is poor or absent, the unconsciousness is deeper and the risk is correspondingly greater.

Every 10 minutes recheck and note the casualty's response to the stimuli of noise (speak loudly into the ear), touch (try to arouse by shaking the shoulders gently) and pain (watch the face, while you pinch the skin), or hand (ankle). In addition, the casualty's breathing, pulse and temperature should be check and recorded.

Aids to Diagnosis

The diagnosis will be based on information from various sources. By taking the history of the incident, asking the casualty for symptoms and examining him/her for signs, it should be possible to make an accurate diagnosis. The following chart is a summary of how to achieve this.

History

History is obtained from surroundings, casualty and bystanders.

History taking

Signs	Symptoms
These are the sensations experienced by the casualty and obtained by asking tactful questions. • Pain • Loss of normal movement • Loss of sensation • Cold • Heat • Thirst • Nausea • Weakness • Dizziness • Faintness • Temporary loss of consciousness • Loss of memory • Sensation of breaking bone	These are noted by first aider using his/her own senses: • Sight • Respiration • Bleeding (type and volume) • Wounds • Foreign bodies • Color of face • Swelling • Bruising • Reflexes • Responses to touch and sound • Incontinence • Vomit • Needle marks • Containers • Hearing • Breathing • Groans • Crepitus • Touch • Dampness (bleeding incontinence) • Temperature • Pulse • Swelling • Deformity • Irregularity • Tenderness • Smell • Breath • Burning

External Clues

If a casualty is unconscious, check their pockets, handbag or briefcase for possible clues. Appointment cards for a hospital or clinic or information cards may reveal that the casualty is on steroids or insulin or is liable to epileptic fits. Lumps of sugar or glucose present may even indicate that the casualty is diabetic ('MedicAlert'). A locket for wrist or neck, a capsule, a neck chain or key ring containing a strip of paper may describe the casualty's condition.

Treatment

Carry out the appropriate treatment for each condition found gently and quickly. It is most important that to reassure and encourage the casualty constantly. Work calmly and efficiently. Pay attention to any remarks or request that the casualty makes, and do not pester with questions. After giving the necessary treatment, place the casualty in the appropriate position and keep a watchful eye until help arrives. Bear in mind your aim is to preserve life, prevent the condition worsening and promote recovery.

To preserve life
- Maintain an open airway by positioning the casualty correctly
- Begin resuscitation, if the casualty is not breathing and the heart is not beating
- Continue treatment until skilled medical aid is available
- Control bleeding

To prevent the condition worsening
- Dress wounds
- Provide comfortable support for any large wounds and fractures
- Place the casualty in the most comfortable position consistent with the requirements of treatment.

To promote recovery
- Relieve the casualty of anxiety and encourage confidence
- Attempt to relieve the casualty of pain and discomfort
- Handle the casualty gently
- Protect the casualty from the cold and wet.

After Treatment

Once the treatment is carried out, the casualty should normally receive attention from a qualified person (doctor or nurse) without undue delay. Depending on the severity of the condition and the availability of skilled help, the following points should be followed:
- Arrange transportation to hospital by ambulance (or by car for minor injuries and arm fractures).
- Handover the casualty to the care of a doctor or nurse at the scene.

- Take the casualty to a nearby house or shelter to await the arrival of the ambulance or doctor.
- Allow the casualty to go home and advise him/her to seek medical advice, if necessary.

> **Note:**
> Never send anyone home who has been unconscious even for a short time or who is in shock; seek medical aid.

Making Report

The casualty should always be accompanied by a brief written report when the care is completed. If necessary, accompany the casualty and prepare personal report. The need to supply complete information cannot be emphasized enough and it should include the following:
- History of the accident or illness
- Brief description of the injury
- The level of responsiveness and any changes
- Any other associate injuries
- The pulse and any changes
- The skin color and any changes
- Blood loss sustained
- Any unusual behavior by the casualty
- Any treatment is given and when?

Informing Relatives

Send a tactful message to the casualty's home stating what has happened and where he/she has been taken if this has not already been done by the police or other authority attending the incident. If the casualty is unconscious or unable to provide contact information about his/her relatives, look for a diary or donor card, which may give the relevant details (refer topic 'external clues').

Property

Take care of any property belonging to the casualty and hand it over to the police or ambulance personnel.

Removing Clothing

Sometimes, it is necessary to remove clothing in order to expose injuries, make an accurate diagnosis or conduct a proper treatment. This should be done with the minimum of disturbance to the casualty and clothing should only be remove as much as is actually necessary. Clothing should not be damaged unnecessarily. If very tight underclothing such as a girdle has to be cut, do this along the seams, if it is possible. Maintain sufficient privacy.

Removing a coat or jacket

Raise the casualty and slip the garment over his/her shoulders. Bend his/her arm on the sound side and remove the coat from that side first. Then slip the injured arm out of its sleeve, keeping the arm straight if possible. If necessary, slit up the seam on the casualty's injured side.

Removing a shirt or vest

Remove a coat, if necessary slit it down the front or side.

Removing trousers

Pull them down from the waist to reveal the casualty's thigh or raise the trouser leg to expose the calf and knee; if necessary slit up the inside seam.

Removing boots or shoes

Support the ankle, undo or cut any laces and carefully remove the shoe. If the casualty is wearing long boots, that will not unfasten, carefully slit them down the back seam with a sharp knife.

Removing socks

If these are difficult to remove insert first two fingers between the sock and the leg. Raise the socks and cut it between the fingers with scissors.

Removing crash helmets

Whether or not you remove a protective helmet, such as motor cycle crash helmet, depends on the situation and condition of the casualty. It is best left on and should only be removed, if the casualty's condition warrants it. If possible, the helmet should be removed by the casualty. A full face helmet that encloses the head and face should only be removed, if it obstructs breathing, if the casualty is vomiting or if there are severe head injuries.

Removing an open face helmet

Unfasten or cut through the chinstrap, if necessary. Take pressure off the head by forcing the sides apart, then lift the helmet upwards and backwards.

Removing a full face helmet

To remove it safely, two people are needed, one to support the casualty's head and neck, while the other lifts the helmet:
- Tilt the helmet back and gently lift until it is clear of the chin.
- Tilt the helmet forward to pass over the base of the skull, then lift it straight off.

REVIEW QUESTIONS

LONG ESSAYS

1. Define first aid. Explain briefly about the scope of first aid.
2. Enumerate principles of first aid. Describe the role of first aider during management of a case.
3. Describe the various action that needs to be taken at an emergency situation.

SHORT ESSAYS

1. Golden rules of first aid.
2. Steps to be taken while assessing unconscious patient.
3. List of information to be included in incident report.
4. Steps to be followed during examination of spine.
5. General rules to be followed while calling for assistance.

Essential Body Parts: Structure and Functions

CHAPTER 2

CHAPTER OUTLINE

- Musculoskeletal System
- Respiratory System
- Digestive System
- Circulatory System
- Endocrine System
- Sensory Organs
- Excretory System
- Reproductive System
- Nervous System
- Integumentary System

INTRODUCTION

The human body consist of extracellular components and live cells, arranged into tissues, organs, and systems. The systems that make up the human body each perform a different role, essential for the well-being of the individual. If one system malfunctions, the effects could spread to other systems and significantly impair the body's capacity to function normally. The smallest independent units of living matter in the human body are called cells, and tissues are made up of cells with a similar structure and function. Organs have evolved to perform a certain purpose and are composed of many types of tissue. Systems are made up of a number of organs and tissues that work together to support one or more of the body's survival needs.

To be effective while delivering emergency care, a first aider must be aware of the basic structure and functions of all vital body parts.

The human body system includes (**Fig. 2.1**):

- ❖ Respiratory system
- ❖ Digestive system
- ❖ Circulatory system
- ❖ Endocrine system
- ❖ Sensory organs
- ❖ Musculoskeletal system
- ❖ Excretory system

CHAPTER 2: Essential Body Parts: Structure and Functions

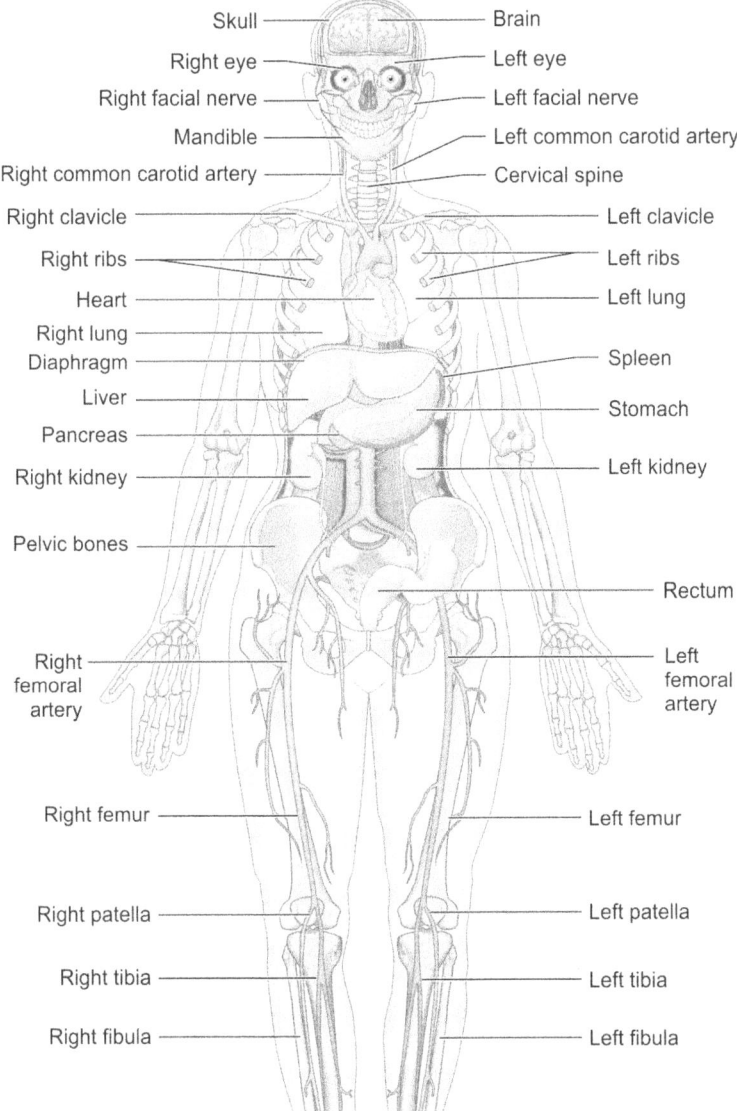

Fig. 2.1: Anatomy of human.

- ❖ Reproductive system
- ❖ Nervous system
- ❖ Integumentary system.

MUSCULOSKELETAL SYSTEM

The musculoskeletal system consists of the bones of the skeleton, their joints and the skeletal (voluntary) muscles that move the body.

Bones

Types of Bone

- Long bones
- Short, irregular, flat and sesamoid bones.

Functions of Bone

- Provide body framework.
- Provide attachment to muscles and tendons.
- Allows movement of the body.
- Protects organs of the body.
- Storage for minerals.

Parts of Bone

- **Head and face:** Skull, two cheek bones and lower jaw bone.
- **Body:** Backbone or spine, the ribs and breast bone.
- **Upper limbs:** Arm, forearm (long bones), palm (short bones).
- **Hip:** The pelvis.
- **Lower limbs:** Thigh and leg—long bones, feet—short bones.

Skull

The skull has a base upon which the brain rests and a vault that surrounds and covers it. The joints between the skulls are immovable in mature skull. The bones of the skull includes **(Fig. 2.2)**:

- **1 frontal bone:** Bone of the forehead.
- **2 parietal bones:** Bones that form the sides and roof of the skull.
- **2 temporal bones:** Bones that lie one on each side of the head.
- **1 occipital bone:** Bones that forms the back of the head and part of the base of the skull.
- **1 sphenoid bone:** Bone that occupies the middle portion of the base of the skull.
- **1 ethmoid bone:** Bones that occupies the anterior part of the base of the skull and helps to form the orbital cavity.

Injury to the head causes bleeding from blood vessels inside the closed box; the blood is unable to escape and gets collected and presses the soft brain tissue. This leads to headache, irritability,

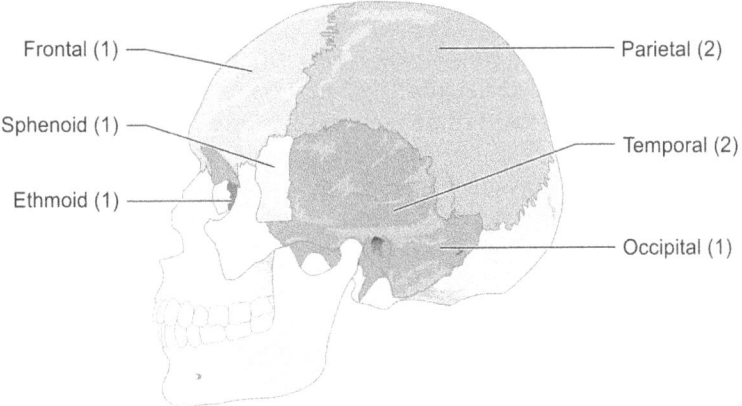

Fig. 2.2: Anatomy of skull: 8 cranial bones.

unconsciousness and may cause death. To avoid this it is important to place all persons of head injury under care of medical supervision at the earliest.

Face

The skeletal of the face is formed by 13 bones. It includes:
- **2 zygomatic (cheek) bones:** These bones fuse before birth and form the prominences of the cheeks and part of the floor and lateral walls of the orbital cavities.
- **1 maxilla:** Fuse before birth and it includes the upper jaw bone.
- **2 nasal bones:** They form the bridge of the nose.
- **2 lacrimal bones:** Two small bones that form part of the medial walls of the orbital cavities.
- **1 vomer:** Extend from the middle hard palate to form inferior of nasal septum.
- **2 palatine bones:** L shape bones that form the posterior part of hard palate.
- **2 inferior conchae:** Scroll-shaped bone, which forms part of the lateral wall of the nasal cavity and projects into it below the middle concha.
- **1 mandible:** This is also called as the lower jaw, the only movable bone of the skull.
- **Hyoid bone:** This is an isolated horseshoe-shaped bone lying in the soft tissues of the neck just above the larynx and below the mandible. This does not coherent with any other bones.

Vertebral Column

The vertebral column consist of 26 bones. The first seven vertebrae, in the neck, form the cervical spine, the next 12 vertebrae are the thoracic spine and the next five the lumbar spine, the lowest vertebra of which articulates with the sacrum. In case of any displacement of the vertebra the spinal cord is pressed or cut causing paralysis extremely important to handle with care all persons who have suffered severe injury to their back or neck.

Movement of vertebral column
- **Flexion:** Bending forward.
- **Extension:** Bending backward.
- **Lateral flexion:** Bending to the side.
- Rotation

> **Note:**
> Understanding movement of vertebral column will help the first aider during movement/transfer of casualty.

Thoracic Cage

It includes the ribs and breast bone (sternum). In sternum the bones can be felt in the middle of the front of the chest. There are 12 pairs of ribs which are elongated curved bones. The thoracic cage protects the heart and the lungs. Any injury of the rib should be taken seriously and requires urgent hospitalization.

Appendicular Skeleton

The appendicular skeleton consist of:
- **Shoulder girdle with the upper limbs:** Upper limb join the trunk of the body through the shoulder gridle.
  - *Clavicle (collar bone):* Extends from sternum to the shoulder.
  - *Scapula (shoulder blade):* Flat triangular-shaped bone situated close to the ribs on the posterior chest wall.
  - *Humerus:* Bones of the upper limb. The head of humerus sits within the glenoid cavity of the scapula, forming the shoulder joint.
  - *Ulna and radius:* Bones of the forearm. They are two parallel bones that articulate with the humerus at the elbow joint.
  - *Carpal (wrist) bones:* Eight carpal bones arranged in two rows of four.

- *Metacarpal bones (bones of the hand):* They are five bones that form the palm of the hand.
- *Phalanges (finger bones):* There are 14 phalanges, three in each finger and two in the thumb. They articulate with the metacarpal bones and with each other, by hinge joints.
- ❖ **Pelvic girdle with the lower limbs:** The lower limb forms a joint with the trunk at the pelvic girdle.
  - *Innominate (hip) bones:* Each hip bone consists of three fused bones—the ilium, ischium and pubis.
  - *Pelvis:* The pelvis is formed by the hip bones, the sacrum and the coccyx.
  - *Femur (thigh bone):* The femur is the longest and heaviest bone of the body with a spherical head and fits into the acetabulum.
  - *Tibia (shin bone):* The medial of the two lower leg bones is called the tibia. The end part of the tibia form the ankle joint.
  - *Fibula:* The fibula is the long slender lateral bone in the leg. This helps to stabilize ankle joint.
  - *Patella (knee cap):* Triangular-shaped sesamoid bone associated with the knee joint.
  - *Tarsal (ankle) bones:* It articulates with the tibia and fibula at the ankle joint. The seven tarsal bones forming the posterior part of the foot (ankle) are the talus, calcaneus, navicular, cuboid and three cuneiform bones.
  - *Metatarsals (bones of the foot):* They articulate with the tarsal bones and at their distal ends, with the phalanges. It includes five bones.
  - *Phalanges (toe bones):* There are 14 phalanges, with two in the big toe (the hallux) and three in each of the remaining toes, grouped similarly to the way the fingers' phalanges are arranged.

Fractures

- ❖ **Simple:** The bone ends do not protrude through the skin.
- ❖ **Compound:** The bone ends protrude through the skin.
- ❖ **Pathological:** Fracture of a bone weakened by disease.

Joints

Joint is the area where two bones meet together or come together. The main function of the joint is it helps in movement and flexibility of the joint. Types of joints includes:
- ❖ Fibrous joints

- ❖ Cartilaginous joints
- ❖ **Synovial joints:** Shoulder joints, elbow joints, proximal and distal radioulnar joints, wrist joint.
- ❖ **Joints of the hands and fingers:** Hip joint, knee joint, ankle joint.
- ❖ Joints of the feet and toes.

Skeletal Muscles

The muscles consist of specialized cells called fibers. It consists of smooth, cardiac and skeletal muscles. The skeletal muscles are under voluntary control and they are attached to the bones. The skeletal muscles contracts when stimulated by a nerve fibers and stops when nerve stimulation stops. The junction that connects the nerve and muscles is called as neuromuscular junction. When a body moves, the muscles and tendons stretch across at least one point then pulls one bone towards another to contracts.

RESPIRATORY SYSTEM

The respiratory system serves as a pathway for both carbon dioxide excretion and the pathway via which oxygen from the atmosphere enters the body. Between the lungs and the body's cells, blood serves as the O_2 and CO_2 transport mechanism.

Internal respiration is the exchange of gases between the blood and the cells. **External respiration** is the exchange of gases between the blood and the lungs. The organs of the respiratory system are (**Fig. 2.3**):

- ❖ **Nose:** Inhalation of air, hair follicles prevent entry of foreign pathogens.
- ❖ **Pharynx:** Passage for both food and air is located behind the nasal chamber.
- ❖ **Larynx:** It is called as vocal cords or voice box, use for breathing, swallowing and talking.
- ❖ **Epiglottis:** Prevents entry of food into the windpipe.
- ❖ **Trachea:** Passage for carrying air in and out of lungs.
- ❖ **Two bronchi:** Left and right bronchi. Passage of air from the mouth to the alveoli and vice versa. The bronchi are lined with mucous membrane that acts as barrier from foreign pathogens.
- ❖ **Bronchioles and smaller air passages called alveoli:** Bronchioles branch off from the bronchi like a tree branches. Air is delivered from the bronchioles to alveoli.

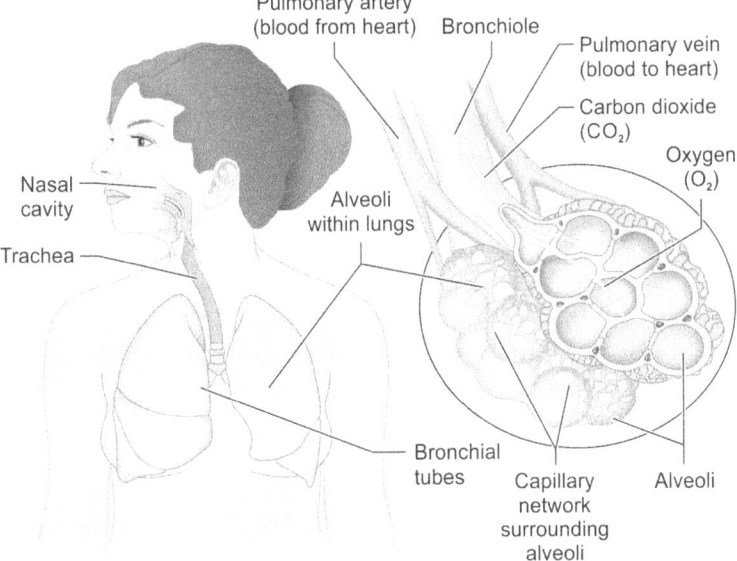

Fig. 2.3: Respiratory system.

- **Two lungs and their coverings, the pleura:** Process of gas exchange takes place, the pleura protects and cushion the lungs.
- **Muscles of breathing:** The intercostal muscles and the diaphragm.

DIGESTIVE SYSTEM

The digestive consist of the alimentary canal and its accessory organs. The digestive system is responsible for the absorption of food that are eaten. The alimentary canal starts at the mouth, passes through the thorax, abdomen and pelvis and ends at the anus. Function of the digestive process is breaking down of foods that are eaten until they are ready for absorption. Parts of alimentary canal includes:

- Mouth
- Pharynx
- Esophagus
- Stomach
- Small intestine
- Large intestine
- Rectum and anal canal

CIRCULATORY SYSTEM

Circulatory system also called as cardiovascular system consist of the heart and various blood vessels. The heart is responsible for pumping of blood, ensuring constant circulation of blood in the body. The blood flows through a blood vessels **(Fig. 2.4)**.

Function

The cardiovascular system makes sure the blood flow never stops. All bodily cells, and its operation is dependent on the constant physiological changes to maintain a sufficient blood flow. When there is an inadequate supply of oxygen and nutrients to the body cells, tissue damage as well as cell death may follow.

Heart

The right side heart pumps blood to the pulmonary circulation and left side pumps blood to the systemic circulation that supplies to rest of the body. The blood is used to excrete tissue wastes, and body cells draw oxygen and nutrients.

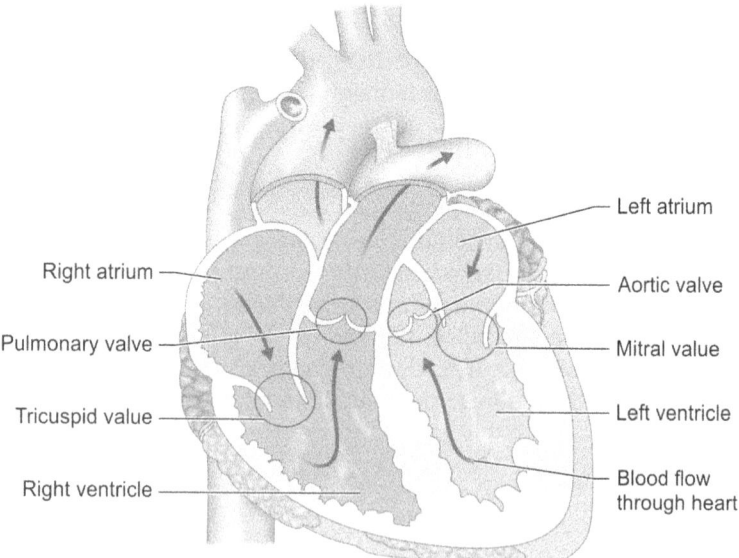

Fig. 2.4: Human heart.

Blood Vessels

Blood vessels are of several types which includes arteries, arterioles, capillaries, venules and veins. They vary in structure, size and function.

- **Arteries and arterioles:** They transport blood away from the heart.
- **Capillaries and sinusoids:** Breaking up of arterioles into minute vessels is called capillaries. Capillaries that are wider and leakier are called sinusoids.
- **Veins and venules:** Veins return blood at low pressure to the heart. The smallest veins are called venules.

ENDOCRINE SYSTEM

Endocrine system consist of group of glands with no physical connection. Endocrine glands are formed by group of secretory cells which are surrounded by an extensive network of capillaries that facilitates diffusion of hormones (chemical messengers) from the secretory cells into the bloodstream. In endocrine system homeostasis of the internal environment is maintained by autonomic nervous system and endocrine system. Hormones of the endocrine glands are carried in the bloodstream to target tissues and organs.

Functions

Endocrine glands release hormones into the bloodstream. They are responsible for cell growth and development, emotions, metabolism, reproduction. Fertility and sexuality.

Glands of the Endocrine System (Fig. 2.5)

- Pituitary gland.
- Thyroid gland.
- Parathyroid gland.
- Adrenal gland.
- Hypothalamus.
- Thymus.
- Pancreas.
- Ovary.
- Testis.

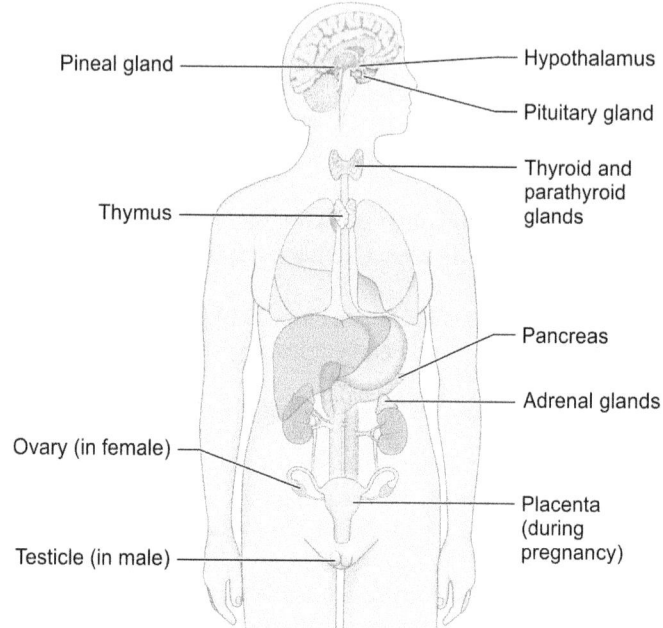

Fig. 2.5: Endocrine system.

SENSORY ORGANS

The special senses of the body includes hearing, sight, smell, taste and sensation.

Ear

Ear is the organ responsible for hearing. Parts of the ear consist of outer ear, middle ear (tympanic cavity) and inner ear. The ear is supplied by the 8th cranial nerve.

Eye

Eye is the organ of sight. The eye is supply by the optic nerve. It consist of sclera, cornea, iris, pupil, lens, retina, optic nerves.

Nasal Cavity

The sense of smell originates in the nasal cavity. It is supply by olfactory nerve.

Tongue

The sense of taste is regulated by taste buds and are widely distributed in the epithelia of the tongue. They consist of small sensory nerve endings of the glossopharyngeal, facial and vagus nerves.

Skin

The body is completely cover by the skin and is responsible for regulation of body temperature. It contains sensory nerve endings that enable discrimination of pain, temperature and touch. It protects the underlying structures from injury and from invasion by microbes.

EXCRETORY SYSTEM

The excretory system is a part of the body that maintain balance between water and electrolytes in the body. The waste products of the body such as nitrogenous compounds—urea, uric acid, excess ions and drugs are excreted in urine which are store in the bladder. This process is called micturition.

The excretory system includes:
- **2 kidneys:** Secretes urine.
- **2 ureters:** Carry the urine from the kidney to the urinary bladder.
- **Urinary bladder:** The urinary bladder collects and stores urine.
- **Urethra:** The site through which urine leaves the body.

Organs associated with kidneys

Right kidney	Left kidney
Superiorly—the right adrenal gland. Anteriorly—the right lobe of the liver, the duodenum and the hepatic flexure of the colon. Posteriorly—the diaphragm, and muscles of the posterior abdominal wall.	Superiorly—the left adrenal gland. Anteriorly—the spleen, stomach, pancreas, jejunum and splenic flexure of the colon. Posteriorly—the diaphragm and muscles of the posterior abdominal wall.

REPRODUCTIVE SYSTEM

The male and female reproductive system differs anatomically and physiologically.

Female Reproductive System

The female reproductive system is responsible for formation of ova and reception of spermatozoa. The female reproductive organs provide suitable environments for fertilization and fetal development. The breast helps in lactation, production of breast milk and provide nourishment for the baby in its early life. Parts of the female reproductive system includes:
* External genitalia (vulva)
* Internal genitalia
* Breasts

Male Reproductive System

The male reproductive system play an important role in production, maturation and storage of spermatozoa. It delivers spermatozoa in semen into the female reproductive tract. Parts of the male reproductive system includes:
* Scrotum
* Testes
* Spermatic cords
* Seminal vesicles
* Ejaculatory ducts
* Prostate glands
* Urethra and penis

NERVOUS SYSTEM

The nervous system coordinate and control vital aspects of the body along with the endocrine system. Compare to the endocrine system the nervous system provides an immediate response. The nervous system consist of:
* **Central nervous system:** Brain and spinal cord
* **Peripheral nervous system:** All nerves outside the brain and spinal cord.

The central nervous system (CNS) receives sensory information about its internal and external environments from afferent nerves. The peripheral nervous system (PNS) includes sensory division and motor division where the motor division are further classified into somatic nervous system and autonomic nervous system (sympathetic and parasympathetic).

Nervous Tissue

- **Neurons:** The neurons generate and transmit nerve impulses.
- **Neuroglia:** Neuroglia are the connective tissue that support the neurons.

INTEGUMENTARY SYSTEM

The integumentary system is the largest organ in the body. The layer of skin includes epidermis and dermis **(Fig. 2.6)**. The accessory structures of the skin consist of glands, hair and nails. The skin color is affected by various factors such as melanin, normal saturation of hemoglobin and excessive levels of bile pigments in blood. Any severe injury to the skin such as burns from heat, cold, electricity, ionizing radiation and corrosive chemicals, including strong acids or alkalis (bases) require immediate medical attention.

Sensory Receptors of Skin

- **Sensory receptor:** Stimulus.
- **Meissner's corpuscle:** Light pressure.
- **Pacinian corpuscle:** Deep pressure.
- **Free nerve ending:** Pain.

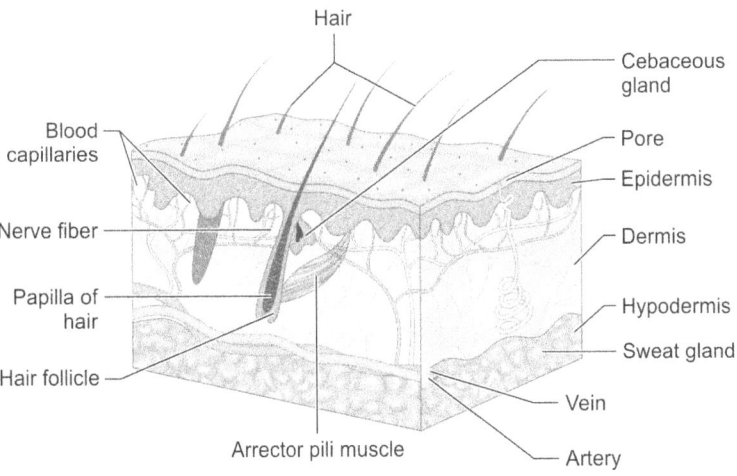

Fig. 2.6: Anatomy of skin.

Functions of the Skin

Protection, regulation of body temperature, formation of vitamin D, cutaneous sensation, absorption, excretion, wound healing.

REVIEW QUESTIONS

LONG ESSAYS

1. Describe musculoskeletal system in detail.
2. Describe parts of respiratory system and their functions.
3. Explain circulatory system.

SHORT ESSAYS

1. Explain in brief appendicular skeleton.
2. Describe parts of the skull.
3. Discuss integumentary system.
4. Describe the sensory organs in details.
5. Explain organs associated with kidneys and their functions.

First Aid Management

SECTION 2

Chapter 3:	Wounds, Hemorrhage and Shock
	3.1: Wounds
	3.2: Hemorrhage
	3.3: Shock
Chapter 4:	Musculoskeletal Injuries
	4.1: Fracture, Muscle Injuries and Dislocation
	4.2: Injuries: Head, Spinal Cord and Others
	4.3: Bandages and Dressings
Chapter 5:	Transportation of Injured Persons
Chapter 6:	Respiratory Emergencies and Basic CPR
	6.1: Respiratory Emergencies
	6.2: Emergency Resuscitation
Chapter 7:	Unconsciousness
Chapter 8:	Foreign Bodies
Chapter 9:	Burns and Scalds
Chapter 10:	Poisoning, Bites and Stings
	10.1: Poisoning
	10.2: Bites and Stings

Chapter 11: Frostbite and Effects of Heat

Chapter 12: Community Emergencies
    12.1: Disaster Management
    12.2: First Aid Kit

Wounds, Hemorrhage and Shock

CHAPTER 3

3.1: WOUNDS

Chapter Outline

- Definition
- Types of Wound
- Abrasions
- Incised Wound
- Lacerated Wound
- Punctured Wound
- Gunshot Wound
- Eye Wounds
- Wound to the Palm of the Hand
- Bruises
- Infected Wounds
- Penetrating Chest Wounds
- Abdominal Wounds
- Crush Injuries
- Ulcers
- Boils

INTRODUCTION

The skin is normally intact. A break or tear in the skin may occur following an accident. The result is a wound. The deeper the wound, the more likely it is to get infected as it cannot be properly cleaned. The appearance of the wound and its likelihood of infection depend on what causes the wound. Would can vary from minor wounds to severe wounds.

Aims of the first aider when dealing with wounds are:
- To stop the bleeding.
- To prevent infection. Injury to the skin may be caused by the following:
  - A cut with a sharp instrument, e.g., knife, glass, stone, etc.
  - A blow with a blunt instrument, e.g., stick, stone, etc.
  - A broken bone whose sharp pierces the skin from inside, usually when open fracture occurs.
- The degree of injury to the skin ranges from an abrasion to a deep wound.

DEFINITION

A break/damage to the integrity of biological tissue, including skin, mucous membranes, and organ tissues.

TYPES OF WOUND

- Abrasions
- Incised wound
- Lacerated wound
- Punctured wound
- Contused wound
- Gunshot wounds
- Eye wounds
- Wound to the palm of the hand
- Bruises
- Infected wounds
- Penetrating chest wounds
- Abdominal wounds
- Crush injuries

Abrasions

An abrasion or graze or scrape are an injury to the superficial layer of the skin that results in disruption of the tissue continuity.

Signs of Abrasions (Fig. 3.1.1)

- Superficial scraping of the skin
- Slight bleeding
- Mild pain
- Redness or swelling may occur

First Aid Measures

- Wash the site with clean boiled water and soap.
- Remove any dirt or other foreign matter.
- Wash with antiseptic lotion and apply gentian violet (GV) paint.
- Apply clean gauze covered with cotton wool padding and bandage.
- Instruct patient to change the dressing once or twice a day.
- Instruct patient to be alert for signs of fever.

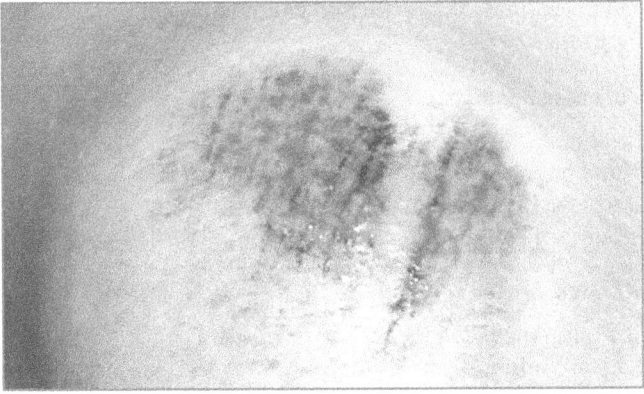

Fig. 3.1.1: Abrasions.

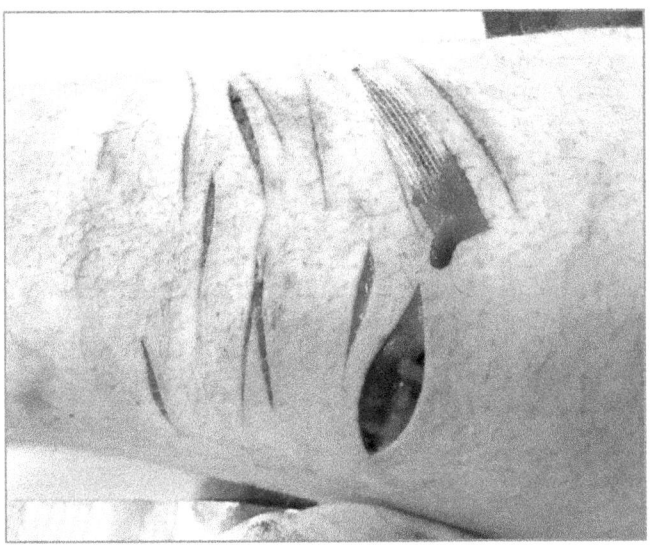

Fig. 3.1.2: Incised wound.

Incised Wound

An incised wound is caused by a sharp cutting instrument **(Fig. 3.1.2)**. Its edges are straight and it is usually accompanied by profuse bleeding, which helps to wash away any germs that might have entered the wound. A deep incised wound may cut through tendons and or arteries.

Signs of Incised Wound
- Bleeding.
- Wound has clear edge.
- Underlying tissue are evenly cut.
- The surface length is greater than depth.

First Aid Measures

Aim is to stop the bleeding as soon as possible:
- Remove clothing around the wound.
- Apply direct pressure to the wound to prevent excessive bleeding.
- Raise the injured area if possible.
- Apply clean gauze covered with cotton wool padding and bandage.
- If the present dressing is soiled with blood do not remove it, add fresh dressing over the top.
- Seek medical attention or take patient to nearby hospital if bleeding does not stop.

Lacerated Wound

A lacerated wound is caused by a blunt instrument. Its edges are ragged and bruising surrounds the wound **(Fig. 3.1.3)**. Usually lacerated wounds do not bleed much and any dirt, which may have entered the wound, is not thoroughly flushed out.

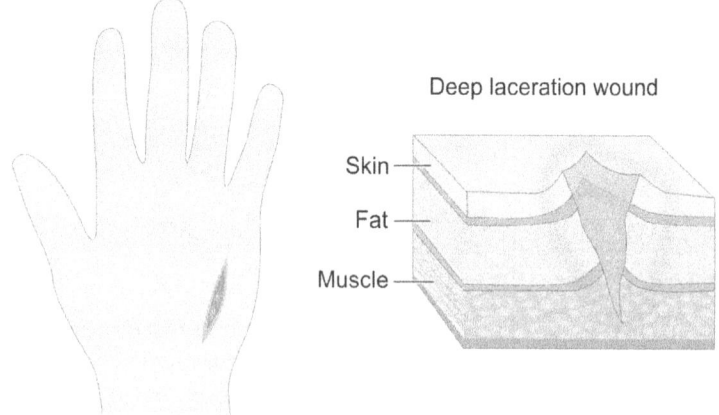

Fig. 3.1.3: Lacerated wound.

Signs of Lacerated Wound
- Pain (mild or severe depending upon the injury).
- Bruising
- Bleeding
- Swelling
- Skin discoloration of the affected area

First Aid Measures
Refer first aid measures of incised wound.

Punctured Wound

A punctured wound is caused by a stab from a knife, needle, nail, bullet, etc., and is often small and deep **(Fig. 3.1.4)**. There is usually little bleeding so that the germs and dirt introduced to the bottom of the wound by the stabbing instrument are not washed out. These wounds are likely to become easily infected and the risk of tetanus is high. Also, because of the depth of these wounds, injury to important structures may be caused.

Signs of Punctured Wounds
- Bleeding
- The appearance of the wound edges depends on type of wound.

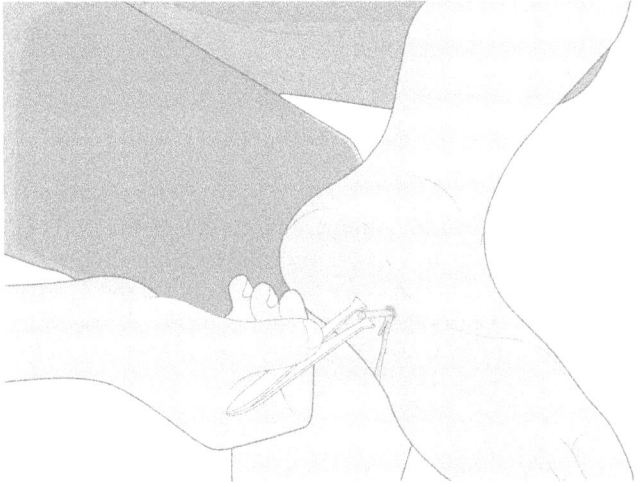

Fig. 3.1.4: Punctured wound.

SECTION 2: First Aid Management

- Signs of shock may be present depending on the severity of the wound and the amount of bleeding.

First Aid Measures

- Handle the injured part gently and as little as possible.
- Sit or lay the patient down and raise the wounded limb.
- Stop the bleeding.
- Treat for shock.
- If the wound is large and will require suturing, apply a dry dressing and transfer the patient to hospital after applying a firm bandage to control the bleeding. Put the arm in a sling or immobilize the leg.
- All punctured wounds of the chest and abdomen after first aid should be referred to the doctor.
- If the wound is small and one can deal with it. Proceed as follows:
  - Sit or lay the patient down.
  - Handle the injured part gently.
  - Clean the wound with soap and boiled water. Always clean away from the wound, not towards it. Remove foreign matter.
  - Stop the bleeding using direct pressure.
  - If the wound is small, apply antibiotic ointment and cover with a clean dry dressing.
  - If the edges of the wound need approximation, use adhesive plaster to bring them together. Apply a dry sterile dressing.

Note:
- Do not disturb the blood clots.
- Do not remove any glass unless it is easily wiped away, as its removal may open up a large blood vessel.

Gunshot Wound

Gunshot wound is caused when a missile strikes the body at high speed and can result in serious internal injury. There will be a wound, where a missile enters the body and often a much larger exit wound (**Fig. 3.1.5**). Internal organs, tissues and blood vessels may be damaged during the missile passage through the body. In addition to external bleeding there may be internal bleeding.

First Aid Measures

- The initial action is to clean the wound.
- Apply the ointment and cover the wound with clean gauze.

CHAPTER 3: Wounds, Hemorrhage and Shock

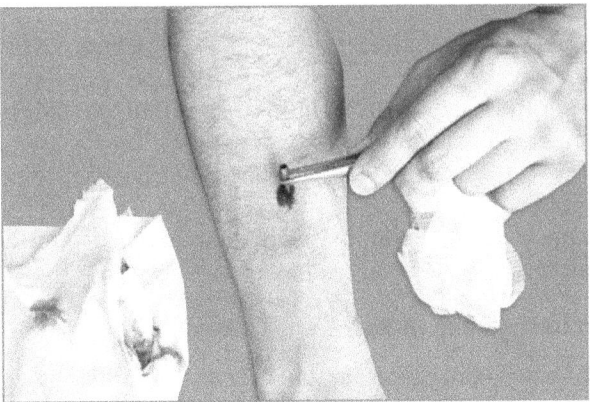

Fig. 3.1.5: Gunshot wound.

- Apply bandages
- Assess the wound for internal injuries
- Take the casualty to nearby hospital.

Eye Wounds

All eye injuries are potentially serious. Even superficial grazes can lead to scarring of the surface of the eye (cornea) on infection, with possible deterioration of eye sight and even permanent blindness. The eye can be cut or bruised by direct flows, broken spectacles, or sharp, clipped fragments of metallic materials, girt or glass, which fly into it.

Symptoms and Signs

- Partial or total loss of vision of the affected eye, even with no visible injury
- Painful, blood shot eye, possibly with a visible wound of eyeball or eyelid
- Loss of blood or clear fluid from the eye wound, possibly with flattening of the normal round contour of the eyeball as the contents leak.

First Aid Measures

Aims: Protect the eye by preventing movement and seek medical aid.
- Lay the casualty down on his/her back. Support his/her head and keep it as still as possible. Do not attempt to remove embedded foreign bodies.

- Ask the casualty to close his/her injured eye and gently cover it with an eye pad or a sterile dressing. Secure it with a bandage or adhesive plaster.
- Instruct the casualty to keep his/her sound eye still because movement will cause the injured eye to move. If necessary, bandage both eyes to prevent unnecessary movement. Reassure the casualty before blindfolding.
- Arrange transportation to hospital, maintaining the treatment position.

Wound to the Palm of Hand

Wounds in the palm can occur, when a person handles broken glass or sharp tools or falls on to sharp objects. Such wounds may bleed profusely and can be accompanied by fractures. If the wound is deep, the nerves and tendons in the hand may be damaged.

Symptoms and Signs
- Pain at the site of the wound
- Bleeding may be profuse
- Loss of sensation and movement in the fingers and hand, if the underlying nerves and tendons are severed.

First Aid Measures

Aims: Control bleeding and arrange immediate transportation to hospital without attempting to remove any embedded foreign bodies.
- To control bleeding, place a sterile dressing or gauze and a clean pad over the wound and apply direct pressure with fingers or thumbs or by casualty if able. If no dressing or pad is available, use an improvised dressing (e.g., a clean handkerchief, a freshly laundered towel, a piece of or a pad of clean paper handkerchief can be used. Improvised dressing should be covered and held in position using whatever materials are available at the time, e.g., a folded scarf).
- Elevate the injured arm above the level of the heart.
- Ask the casualty to maintain pressure by clenching his/her fist over the dressing or pad. If the casualty cannot do this tell to grasp fist of his/her injured hand with other hand.
- Bandage the fists firmly, using the loose ends of the dressing or a folded triangular bandage. Tie off firmly across the bent fingers to maintain pressure.

- Support the arm in an elevation sling and arrange removal to hospital.

Bruises

A bruise consists of internal bleeding, which seeps through the tissues and appears as a discoloration under the skin **(Fig. 3.1.6)**. A heavy fall on fleshy parts of the body, e.g., the buttocks, can result in considerable bruising. A bruise may follow blows, sprains or fractures.

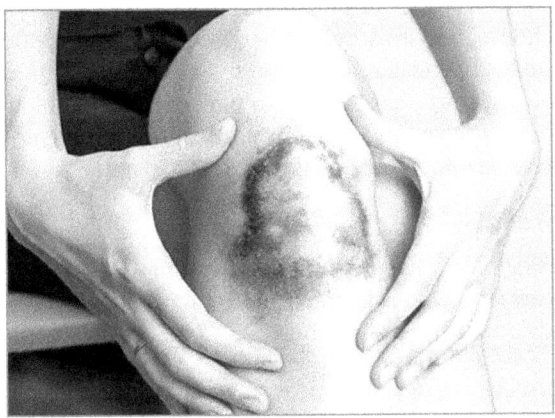

Fig. 3.1.6: Bruise.

Symptoms and Signs
- Pain and swelling in the affected area
- Bluish-purple discoloration at site of injury
- Pattern bruising, in which outlines of the casualty's clothing are seen in the bruise. This is a potentially dangerous sign as it may indicate damage to internal organs.

First Aid Measures
Aims: Slow down blood flow by cooling and gentle compression.

Treatment
- Raise and support the injured part in the position the casualty finds most comfortable.
- Apply a cold compress to the injured area to restrict bleeding and reduce swelling.
- If in doubt about the severity of the injury, seek medical aid.

Infected Wounds

All open wounds will be contaminated by germs, which either come from the cause of the injury, from the air or from the first aider's breath or fingers. Some particles of dirt may be carried away from the damaged tissue by bleeding. Any harmful germs, which remains are usually destroyed by the white cells in the blood, and wound then stays clean and healthy.

Normal first aid for wounds includes prevention of infection. However, any wound, which has not begun to heal properly after about 48 hours, may be infected because dirt, dead tissue, foreign bodies and/or bacteria may still be present. If infection develops, it can have serious consequences. It may enter in the blood system and subsequently spread to other parts of the body, permanently destroying tissue and occasionally leading to death.

Symptoms and Signs
- Increasing pain and soreness in the wound
- Increased surrounding parts with a feeling of heat
- Pus may ooze from the wound
- Fever, sweating, thirst, shivering and lethargy, if the infection is severe
- Swelling and tenderness in the glands, in the neck, armpits or groin
- Faint read trails may be seen on the surface of the inside of the arms or legs leading towards lymph glands

First Aid Measures
Aim is to seek medical aid.
- Dress wound with a prepared sterile dressing and secure with a bandage.
- Elevate the injured part and immobilize especially, if swollen.
- Seek medical aid.

Tetanus Infection (Lock Jaw)
Tetanus infection is particularly dangerous infection results from tetanus germs in a wound, which produce a toxic substance. This spreads into the body's nerves, causing severe muscular spasm, particularly in the jaw, hence the name 'lock jaw'. It is difficult condition to treat and if not treated at an early stage, can lead to

the death of the casualty. Every wound carries the risk of tetanus infection, but the disease is preventable by immunization. Everyone should be inoculated against tetanus regularly and should always ask a wounded casualty how recently inoculation was given. Any casualty with a wound who has never had an 'antitetanus' injection or whose last infection was more than 3 years ago, should be referred to medical advice.

Penetrating Chest Wounds

The rib cage protects not only the heart, lungs and major blood vessels in the chest cavity above the diaphragm, but also the liver and spleen below the diaphragm in the upper abdominal cavity. A wound to the front or back of the chest, which penetrates into the chest allows air to enter the space occupied by the lungs, this interfering with breathing. In these injuries, the lung on the affected side collapses, even if it is not punctured. Air in the chest cavity impairs the action of the sound lung and, sometimes, of the heart. The amount of oxygen reaching the bloodstream may be insufficient and asphyxia may result. A wound to the front or back of the lower chest may penetrate into the abdominal cavity and give rise to severe internal bleeding.

Symptoms and Signs

- Casualty may have pain in the chest and may have an acute sense of alarm
- Difficulty in breathing; breaths are shallow due to air in the chest cavity
- Blueness of the mouth, nail beds and skin (cyanosis) indicating the onset of significant asphyxia
- Bright red, frothy blood may be coughed up
- The sound of air being sucked into the chest may be heard when the casualty is breathing in
- Blood-stained liquid bubbling from the chest wound during breathing out
- Symptoms and signs of shock.

First Aid Measures

Aim is to ease breathing by immediately sealing the wound. Arrange immediate transportation to hospital.

Treatment

- Immediately seal open wound with palm or the casualty's if possible.
- Place the casualty in a half-sitting position with his/her head and shoulders supported; turn the body towards the injured side so the sound lung is upper most.
- Pressure the casualty.
- Gently cover the wounds with a sterile dressing as soon as possible.
- If possible, form an airtight seal by covering the dressing with a plastic sheet or metal foil. Secure and seal the edges of the dressing with layers of adhesive tape, strapping and/or bandage.
- Support the arm on the injured side in an elevation sling and make the casualty as comfortable as possible.
- Check breathing rate, pulse and level of responsiveness at 10-minute intervals. Look for evidence of internal bleeding.
- If the casualty becomes unconscious, open airway and check breathing. Complete CAB of resuscitation, if requires and place in the recovery position with his/her uninjured side upper most.
- Arrange urgent transportation to hospital. Transport as a stretcher case, maintaining the treatment position.
- If a foreign body is present give first aid as for foreign body.

Abdominal Wounds

Wounds of the abdominal wall may be caused by sharp instruments or by missiles. A deep wound of the abdominal wall is serious not only because of the external bleeding, but also because the underlying organs may have been punctured or lacerated, leading to severe internal bleeding and possible infection. Part of the intestine may also be protruding from the wound.

Symptoms and Signs

- General abdominal pain
- Bleeding and associated wounds (which may only be a small puncture) in the abdominal area
- Part of the intestine may be visible in or protruding from the wound
- Casualty may be vomiting
- Symptoms and signs of shock.

First Aid Measures

Aims is to protect wound to minimize infection and arrange immediate transportation to hospital.

1. Lay the casualty on his/her back with knees bent up to prevent the wound gaping and to reduce strain on the injured area. Support the knees.
2. Apply sterile dressing or gauze and a clean pad over the wound and secure with a bandage or adhesive strapping.
3. To minimize shock, if shock present and treatment to shock.

> **Note:**
> Do not remove protruding objects or do not give the casualty anything by mouth.

4. Check breathing rate and pulse at 10-minute intervals. Look for evidence of internal bleeding.
5. If the casualty coughs or vomits, support his/her abdomen by pressing gently on the dressing to prevent protrusion of the intestines from the wound.
6. If he/she becomes unconscious, open his/her airway and check breathing. Complete the CAB of resuscitation, if required and support his/her abdomen when placing his/her in recovery position.
7. Arrange urgent transportation to hospital. Transport as a stretcher case, maintaining the treatment position.

If part of the intestine protrudes from the wound. Do not touch the protruding intestines:
- Cover with a sterile dressing or clean cloth secured with a bandage.
- If the casualty coughs or vomits, support the wound as in step 5.
- Position and treat the casualty as above.

Crush Injuries

Crush injuries commonly occur in earthquakes, bomb incidents, mining accidents and demolition work. Prolonged crushing of a mass of muscles, e.g., in the thigh, leads to shock because of the blood loss into the tissues after the casualty has been freed. Toxic substances released by the damaged muscles are introduced into the casualty's circulation and may lead to kidney failure. This sequence is known as 'the Crush syndrome', because of the danger of kidney failure in all cases where a casualty has been trapped for longer than 1 hour, call the emergency services immediately and do not attempt to release him/her.

Symptoms and Signs

- Crushed limb may be tingling or numb
- Swollen and hard tissue around injured part because serum has poured into the area
- Bruising and formation of blisters at the site of injury
- Crushed or trapped limb will be cool, pale and pulseless, if arteries are compressed
- Symptoms and signs of fracture
- Symptoms and signs of shock

First Aid Measures

Aims is to prevent damage to the kidneys; arrange immediate medical assistance, if the casualty has been trapped for more than 1 hour.

If trapped for less than 1 hour:
- Release the casualty as quickly as possible.
- Elevate the limb if the injuries allow to do so.
- Control any bleeding and treat any wounds.
- Immobilize any fractures, if present.
- Position as for treatment of shock and remove to hospital if necessary.

Note:
Record time of release and duration of crushing.

If trapped for more than 1 hour:
- Do not attempt to release the casualty.
- Reassure and make his/her as comfortable as the circumstances permit.
- Call for medical assistance and emergency services.

Ulcers

An ulcer is formed when there is loss of tissue at the surface of the skin. The loss tissue results from an infection, which destroys the cells. Ulcers occur after injury, infection or because of a faulty diet. They also occur in patients suffering from chronic diseases, such as leprosy, syphilis, tuberculosis or filariasis.

Types

1. **Acute ulcer:** The ulcer is painful, tender and discharges serum. Later on pus forms and the ulcer has a foul smell. Spreads of dead tissue may be seen. The edges of such an ulcer are swollen. Acute ulcers arise from an infected cut or from a skin infection.
2. **Chronic ulcer:** It accompanies chronic diseases, malnutrition, underlying bone infection and neglected acute ulcers. These ulcers have a foul smell, their edges are raised and spreading and they are painful.

If patient has ulcer, go through the following checklist **(Table 3.1.1)**.

Table 3.1.1: Checklist to treat patient with ulcer.

Checklist	Acute ulcer	Chronic ulcer
Duration	Day	Week or month
Constitutional symptoms	No	Yes
Signs of malnutrition	No	May be
Depth of ulceration	Superficial	Deep

Treatment for Acute Ulcer

- Hot fomentation
- Dressing with GV paint. If possible, change twice a day.
  - If better—continued dressings till it heals.
  - If no better—refer to doctor.

A chronic ulcer should always be referred to the doctor to exclude a chronic disease.

Boils

A boil is an infection of the skin caused by the germs entering the skin glands. Each boil begins as a small firm, painful swelling and if it is neglected, or badly treated it develops into an abscess.

Signs and Symptoms

A boil is one of the commonest conditions, which one is likely to see in the home. The condition occurs more commonly in children, especially children, who do not bathe frequently and whose skin is dirty. Bad nutrition and diabetes can also lead to boils. The signs and symptoms of a boil are:

- Swelling.
- Redness of the affected area.

- ❖ Tenderness of the affected area.
- ❖ Pain, sometimes throbbing pain. These local symptoms may be accompanied by general symptoms mainly:
  - ♦ Fever
  - ♦ Headache

Treatment

Apply hot fomentations with magnesium sulphate solution to the affected area.

> **Note:**
> - If treatment is started early, the process may be stopped and abscess formation prevented.
> - If a person who suffers from frequent boils should be seen by a doctor to exclude chronic disease.

REVIEW QUESTIONS

LONG ESSAYS

1. List the types of wounds and explain punctured wounds in details.
2. Distinguish between abrasions and incised wounds. Describe their first-aid measures.
3. List first aider aims for management of wounds. Explain crush injuries in details.

SHORT ESSAYS

1. First aid for gunshot wounds.
2. First aid measures for abdominal wounds.
3. First aid measures for penetrating chest wounds.
4. Explain bruises.
5. First aid measures for eye wounds.

3.2: HEMORRHAGE

CHAPTER OUTLINE

- Definition
- Classification
- Common Signs and Symptoms
- First Aid Measures of Hemorrhage
- General Guidelines and Management
- Severe External Bleeding
- Internal Bleeding
  - Scalp Wound
- Nose Bleed
- Bleeding from the Ear
- Bleeding from the Mouth
- Bleeding from Varicose Veins
- Vaginal Bleeding
- Miscarriage

INTRODUCTION

Hemorrhage or bleeding may vary in intensity from severe to slight. Severe hemorrhage comes from a torn artery or torn vein or both combined. Many large arteries and veins lie close together and are frequently injured together. Slight hemorrhage comes usually from injured capillaries and may flow in a continuous stream as merely ooze from all parts of the wound. There are different types of bleeding, i.e., arterial, venous and capillary. Each is named after the type of blood vessel damaged. Major arterial bleeding is the most serious and must always be treated first. Capillary bleeding is always present. However, in some wounds arterial and venous bleeding will both be evident.

DEFINITION

Hemorrhage is defined as the excess loss of blood due to rupture of blood vessels.

CLASSIFICATION (FLOWCHART 3.2.1)

- **Accidental hemorrhage:** Hemorrhage that occurs in road accidents and industrial accidents. It is of two types:
  1. *Primary hemorrhage:* Occurs immediately after the accident.
  2. *Secondary hemorrhage:* Occurs few hours after the accident.

Flowchart 3.2.1: Classification of hemorrhage.

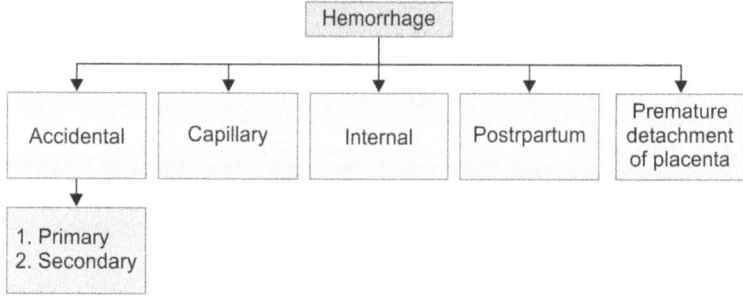

- ❖ **Capillary hemorrhage:** Hemorrhage that occurs due to rupture of blood vessels, especially capillaries, e.g., cerebral hemorrhage.
- ❖ **Internal hemorrhage:** Hemorrhage that occurs in the viscera.
- ❖ **Postpartum hemorrhage:** Severe bleeding that occurs immediately after labor.
- ❖ **Hemorrhage due to premature detachment of placenta:** The placenta is detached from the uterus of mother before the due date of delivery causing severe hemorrhage.

COMMON SIGNS AND SYMPTOMS OF HEMORRHAGE

- ❖ Decrease blood pressure
- ❖ Decrease stroke volume
- ❖ Tachycardia
- ❖ Grayish pallor color of skin
- ❖ Cyanosis
- ❖ Cold and clammy skin
- ❖ Decrease capillary pressure
- ❖ Decrease urinary output
- ❖ Hypoxia
- ❖ Restlessness, anxiety and increased motor activity.
- ❖ Fainting
- ❖ It can lead to brain damage

FIRST AID MEASURES OF HEMORRHAGE/BLEEDING

The main objective is to stop/control bleeding

Methods for Controlling Blood Loss

The principle of controlling blood loss is to restrict blood flow to the wound and therefore encourage clotting. Bleeding is control by applying pressure and elevation. Pressure can be applied in two ways:

1. **Direct pressure:** To stop bleeding, apply direct pressure immediately on the wound. This direct pressure flattens the blood vessels in the area and helps to slow down the flow of blood, so that clots can form. Pressure has to be maintained 5-15 minutes because it takes time to halt the flow of blood. If the wound is gaping, squeeze the edges together gently, but firmly. Ask casualty to apply direct pressure if they are capable.

   Direct pressure should be done in the following ways:
   - Cover the wound with a sterile dressing and apply direct pressure with thumb and/or fingers.
   - Lay the casualty down in a suitable and comfortable position. Raise the injured part as high as possible, support it.
   - Apply sterile dressing and sufficient padding to extend well beyond the edges of a wound, and in case of a limb, to encircle it.
     - If no sterile dressing is available, an improvised dressing can be made from any suitable clean material.
     - If bleeding continues, apply further padding and bandage firmly. Do not remove the original dressing, as this may disturb clots and restart the bleeding.
   - Press the padding down and secure with a bandage tied firmly enough to control bleeding, but not so tight as to cut off circulation and immobilize the injured part.

2. **Indirect pressure:** If bleeding cannot be controlled by direct pressure or if it is impossible to apply direct pressure successfully (for example, if there are severe lacerations), one may be able to control it by applying indirect pressure at the appropriate pressure point. Indirect pressure can be used only to control arterial bleeding from a limb. Indirect pressure is done by compressing an artery against an underlying bone to flatten it and prevent the flow of blood beyond that point. However, since this cuts off the supply of blood to the tissues of the entire limb, this method should only be used as a last resort and must not be applied for longer than 15 minutes.

SECTION 2: First Aid Management

GENERAL GUIDELINES AND MANAGEMENT OF HEMORRHAGE

- Calm the casualty and call for ambulance.
- Remove any non-embedded foreign objects like glass, stones, etc., if easily visibile.
- Handle the injured part as gently as possible.
- Make the patient lie down.
- First aid providers must control external bleeding by applying direct pressure **(Fig. 3.2.1)**.
- Indirect pressure and elevation should not be applied first.
- Tourniquets should be used in extraordinary circumstances (such as disaster, war-like settings, isolated places, or by particularly trained first responders) when direct pressure fails to stop life-threatening bleeding or is impossible (e.g., many injuries, inaccessible wounds, multiple victims).
- If a tourniquet needs to stay in place for an extended period of time, cooling the distal limb should be taken into consideration.
- If the wound is on a limb and there are no broken bones, raise the limb. If bleeding continues, do not take off the original dressing, but add more pads and bandage firmly

Severe External Bleeding

The bleeding occurs most often after a deep incision or laceration in the skin. In major external bleeding, always remember that if the

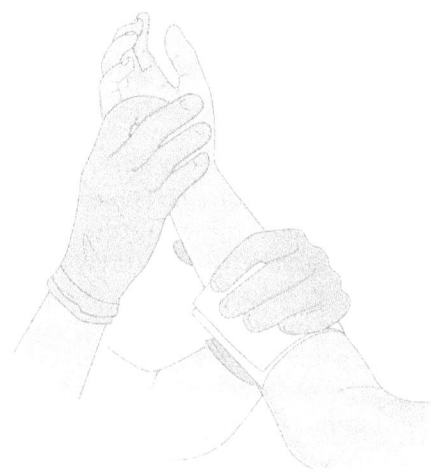

Fig. 3.2.1: Direct pressure of wound with elevation.

casualty is not breathing, begin artificial ventilation. If he/she is unconscious, maintain an open airway, complete the circulation, airway and breathing (C-A-B) of resuscitation, and then treat the bleeding. Otherwise, treat the casualty in the position, which makes blood control most effective.

Signs and Symptoms

- Evidence of major external blood loss
- Shock
- Casualty complains of thirst
- Breathing may become shallower, sometimes accompanied by yawning and sighing
- In more severe cases, deep sighing or gasping (air hunger) may occur
- Vision may be blurred
- Unconsciousness may be possible

First Aid Measures

Aims: Control bleeding and minimize infection.

Management

- Put on disposable gloves if available.
- Cut or remove garments to reveal the wound.
- Over a sterile dressing, non-fluffy clean pad, or clean piece of fabric, apply direct pressure to the wound with the fingers or palm **(Fig. 3.2.1)**.
- Reduce blood loss by raising and supporting the damaged limb above the level of the victim's heart.
- If there is a chance of a fracture, handle the limb extremely lightly; if a blanket is available, assist the victim in laying down so they can avoid the cold.
- Support legs so that they are above the level of the casualty's heart (to avoid shock).
- If additional bleeding occurs, place a second dressing on top of the first one and secure it with a bandage that is snug enough to maintain pressure but not so snug as to restrict circulation.
- Do not remove both dressings if blood seeps through this one; instead, apply a new one, making sure to apply pressure precisely where the bleeding is occurring; Examine the circulation outside of the bandage.

- Support the injured part in a raised position using a sling and/or bandaging; call for medical help.
- Monitor and record the casualty's vital signs—responsiveness level, pulse, and breathing. Watch for signs of shock.

Internal Bleeding

Internal bleeding may occur following an injury such as fracture, crush or penetrating injury, or because of a medical condition such as bleeding, stomach ulcer, external organs, the spleen and liver, for example, can be damaged by blows to the body, although there may be no external evidence. Internal bleeding may be more serious than external bleeding. The blood is not actually lost from the body, it is lost from the circulatory system and the vital organs become starved of oxygen. Blood collecting internally may also cause complications, if it presses on vital structures. For example, blood inside the skull can compress the brain causing loss of consciousness; bleeding inside the chest may prevent the lungs expanding.

Signs and Symptoms

These will vary according to the amount of bleeding and the rate at which blood is lost.
- Pain and tenderness around the affected area; swelling and tension may be left, as in the thigh.
- Similar with symptoms and signs of shock.
- Increase pulse rate.
- Breathing may be shallow.
- Casualty may become restless and talkative.
- Casualty may complain of thirst.
- Blood may appear from one of the body's orifices.

First Aid Measures

Aims: Arrange urgent transportation to hospital, because it is not usually possible to control internal bleeding using first aid.

Management

- Lay the casualty down with head low and to one side, to ensure a good blood supply to brain. Advise not to move.
- If the injuries allow, raise legs to aid the return of blood flow to the vital organs.
- Loosen any constricting clothing around neck, chest and waist.

- Check breathing rate, pulse, level of responsiveness at 10 minute intervals and record it.
- Examine the casualty for other injuries and treat as necessary.
- If he/she becomes unconscious, open airway and check breathing. Complete the 'CAB' of resuscitation', if required and place him/her in the recovery position.
- Keep the casualty covered and place a blanket underneath him/her, if possible.
- Keep a record of any specimen passed or vomited by the casualty. If possible, send samples to the hospital with him/her.
- Arrange urgent transportation to hospital. Transport as a stretcher case, maintaining the treatment position. Do not give the casualty anything by mouth.

Special Forms of Bleeding

There are a number of wounds and special forms of bleeding, where the treatment does not follow the general rules of direct and indirect pressure and/or position of the injured part. Treatment for these wounds are described below in details.

Scalp Wounds

Injuries to the scalp most often occur during falls and are particularly common amongst the elderly, ill or intoxicated. Other causes include road traffic accidents, fights, sporting accidents and falling debris. Scalp wounds can bleed profusely due to the rich supply of blood to the scalp and because the skin covering the skull is normally stretched. When damaged the skin splits open, leaving a gaping wound. This bleeding may appear more alarming than it really is, but the casualty may also have a skull fracture.

Signs and Symptoms
- Pain, tenderness and bleeding of the scalp, possible lifted flap of scalp
- Swelling around the wound
- Possible symptoms and signs of skull fracture
- Signs of brain damage may be evident
- Unconsciousness may develop.

First Aid Measures
Aim: Control bleeding as soon as possible. Arrange transportation to hospital, as all head injuries should be examined by a doctor.

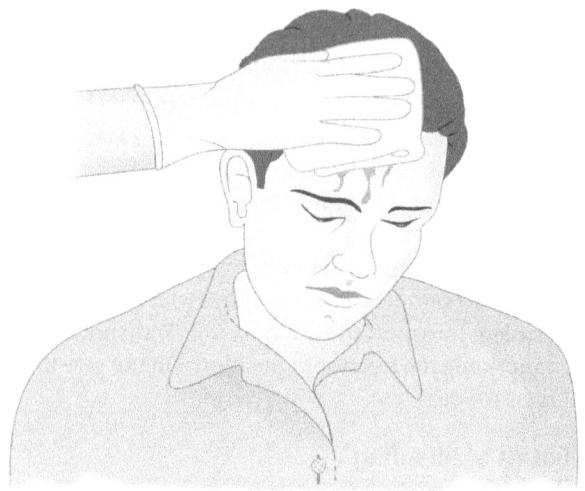

Fig. 3.2.2: Direct pressure on scalp wound.

- Control the bleeding using direct pressure as shown in **Figure 3.2.2**.
- Cover the wound with a sterile or clean dressing or a pad of clean material. Retain with a bandage.
- If the casualty is conscious, carefully and gently lay him/her down with head and shoulders slightly raised.
- Check breathing rate, pulse, level of responsiveness at 10 minute intervals and record it.
- If he/she becomes unconscious, open airway and check breathing. Complete the 'CAB' of resuscitation', if required and place him/her in the recovery position.
- Arrange urgent transportation to hospital. Transport as a stretcher case, maintaining the treatment position

Nose Bleeds (Epistaxis)

Nose bleed is a common condition, usually due to bleeding from the blood vessels inside the nostrils. It may occur after a blow to the nose or better result of sneezing, picking or blowing the nose. However, watery-looking, blood-stained fluid discharge from the nose may be a sign of a fractured skull. Nose bleeds can cause considerable loss of blood and may also cause the casualty to swallow or inhale a great deal of blood. This may cause vomiting or affect breathing.

Signs and Symptoms

- Moderate flow of blood from nose.
- If skull fracture is present, there may be a mixture of blood and clear, watery cerebrospinal fluid.

First Aid Measures (Fig. 3.2.3)

Aim: Safeguard the breathing by preventing inhalation of blood and control bleeding.

- Make the casualty to sit down with head well forward and loosen any tight clothing around neck and chest.
- Advise him/her to breathe through the mouth and to pinch the soft part of nose (be prepared to takeover, if it is tiring for him/her).
- Avoid speech, swallowing, coughing, spitting or sniffing. Allow him/her to dribble and mop it up. Do not let the casualty raise his/her head.
- While the head is still forward, if possible, get the casualty gently to clean around the nose and mouth using a swab (as clean dressing) soaked in lukewarm water. Do not plug the nose.

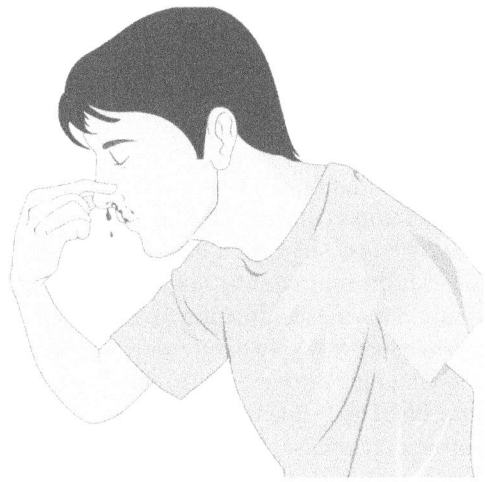

Fig. 3.2.3: First aid for nose bleeding.

- When the bleeding stops, tell the casualty to avoid exertion and not to blow the nose for at least 4 hours, so as not to disturb the clot.
- If even after 30 minutes, the bleeding persists or recurs, seek medical aid.

Bleeding from the Ear

Bleeding from inside the ear canal differs from that found in external ear wounds. It generally occurs when an ear drum ruptures or when a skull fracture is present. A perforated eardrum can result from pushing an object into the ear, falling, while waterskiing, diving or being too near an explosion. Skull fractures are more serious and should be suspected, if blood or clear, watery cerebrospinal fluid mixed with blood is issuing from the ear.

Signs and Symptoms
Eardrum
- Possible pain inside the ear.
- Deafness.
- Moderate flow of blood from the ear.

Within the skull
- History indicating possible skull fracture or other head injury.
- Casualty complains of a headache.
- Small amounts of blood mixed with clear, watery cerebrospinal fluid may be coming from the ear.
- Possible unconsciousness.

First Aid Measures

Aims: Arrange transportation to hospital. If skull fracture is suspected, pay particular attention to the level of responsiveness.

- Place the conscious casualty in a half-sitting position with head inclined towards the injured side, so that blood or fluid can drain.
- Cover the ear with a sterile dressing or similar clean, preferably sterile material. Secure it very lightly with a bandage or adhesive strapping. Do not plug the ear or try to stop the flow from the ear; pressure may build up inside the middle ear.
- Check breathing rate, pulse, level of responsiveness at 10 minute intervals and record it.
- To minimize shock, treat for shock.

CHAPTER 3: Wounds, Hemorrhage and Shock | 63

- If he/she becomes unconscious, open airway and check breathing. Complete the 'CAB' of resuscitation, if required and place him/her in the recovery position.
- Arrange transportation to hospital. Transport as a stretcher case, maintaining the treatment position.

Bleeding from the Mouth

Cuts in tongue, lips or lining of the mouth range from trivial injuries to larger wounds. They are usually caused by the casualty's teeth during falls or a blow to the face. Bleeding may be severe. Bleeding can also occur from the tooth socket after accidental loss of a tooth on sometimes after a dental extraction. Laceration of the gums may occur in association with a fracture of the jaw.

Signs and Symptoms

Bleeding in/or around the mouth or from a tooth socket, pains the affected area.

First Aid Measures

Aims: Safeguard the airway by preventing the inhalation of blood and control bleeding.

- Ask the casualty to sit down with head forward and inclined towards the injured side.
- To control bleeding, place clear dressing over any external wound and tell the casualty to apply direct pressure by squeezing it between his thumb and finger. If a tooth socket is bleeding, place a thick pad of gauze or clear cloth across, not in the socket.

> **Note:**
> This pad must be thick enough to prevent teeth meeting, when the casualty bites.

- The casualty should maintain pressure on the dressing or pad for 10-20 minutes, supporting the chin on his/her hand.
- Allow him/her to dribble out any blood in the mouth, while maintaining pressure; swallowed blood can cause vomiting.
- If bleeding persists after 10-20 minutes, carefully remove dressing or pad, disturbing the clots as little as possible. Renew dressing or pad and continue pressure for a further 10 minutes.

> **Note:**
> This is an exception to the rule that one leaves the first dressing in place when applying a further dressing. Do not wash out the mouth, as this may disturb the clot. Advise the casualty to avoid all hot drinks for 12 hours.

- If the bleeding persists or recurs, seek medical or dental aid.
- If the casualty has lost a tooth and it can be found, place it in a clean container. Seek dental aid as soon as possible and send the tooth with the casualty.

Bleeding in Varicose Veins

The veins in the legs contain valves to keep the blood flowing back to the heart. When these valves deteriorate, they look backwards and the back pressure of the blood causes the veins to become swollen and 'knobbly' or 'varicose'. Such veins can be burst by quite gentle knocks and they bleed severely. If such bleeding is not controlled immediately, the condition can be fatal.

Signs and Symptoms

- Severe external bleeding; blood will be dark red.
- Symptoms and signs of shock.
- Unconsciousness may develop.
- A damaged valve will prevent the correct blood flow.

First Aid Measures

Aims: Control bleeding by elevation and direct pressure. Arrange urgent transportation to hospital.

- Lay the casualty on his/her back and raise the injured leg as high as possible.
- Expose the wound and apply direct pressure by pressing with the fingers or palm of hand over a dressing **(Fig. 3.2.4)**.
- Remove any constricting clothing such as elastic-topped or support stockings, garters or tights, which may be impeding blood flow back to the heart.
- Place a soft pad over the dressing large enough to exert pressure on the whole area around the bleeding varicose vein. Tie a bandage firmly enough to control bleeding, but not so tight as to cut off circulation.

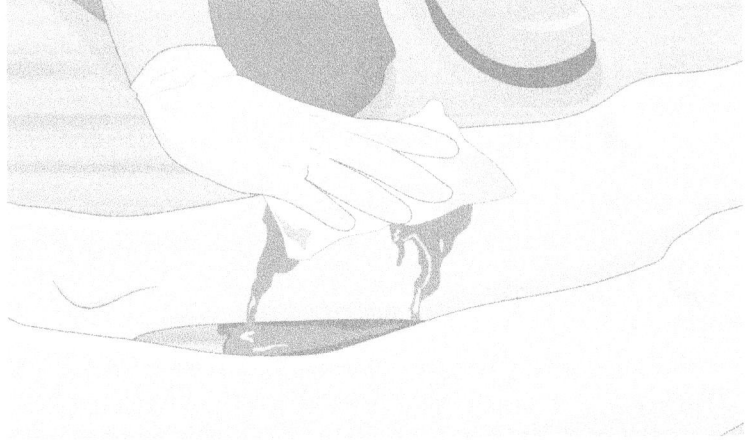

Fig. 3.2.4: Applying direct pressure on bleeding varicose vein.

- If no sterile dressing is available, use an improvised dressing. If bleeding does not stop and bandages are soaked with blood, apply further padding and bandages on top of the original ones.
- Keep the leg raised and supported.
- To minimize shock, treat as on shock.
- Arrange urgent transportation to hospital, maintaining the treatment position.

Vaginal Bleeding

Vaginal bleeding can be severe menstrual bleeding or the result of a miscarriage, internal injury or sexual assault. The history of the condition is essential to the diagnosis of the emergency. It may be due to miscarriage or abortion.

Symptoms

- Moderate to severe bleeding from the vagina.
- Cramp-like pains in the lower abdomen or pelvic area may be present.
- Symptoms and signs of shock may be present.

First Aid Measures

Aims: Reassure the casualty and if in doubt about the severity of the bleeding, arrange transportation to hospital.

- If possible, shift the woman to a place, which has some privacy or arrange for screening. Give her sanitary dressing, if available or a clean towel to be placed over the entrance of the vagina.
- Lay the woman down with head and shoulders raised and knees bent—supported on a blanket (this will relax the abdominal muscles).
- If bleeding continues and is severe, minimize shock by giving treatment for shock. Arrange urgent transportation to hospital, maintaining the treatment position.

Miscarriage

A miscarriage or 'spontaneous abortion' is the loss of the embryo or fetus at any time before the 28th week of pregnancy. It is usually due to abnormality or death of the fetus and is therefore a protective mechanism that avoids the full development and birth of an abnormal baby.

About 20% of all pregnancies end in miscarriage. Although some women may experience a 'threatened' miscarriage involving only slight vaginal bleeding. Complete miscarriages always include the very real danger of severe vaginal bleeding. In complete, miscarriage is a serious condition, because the products of conception are retained in the womb resulting in severe bleeding.

Signs and Symptoms
- Vaginal bleeding; if severe, symptoms and signs of shock may also be present.
- Cramp-like pains in the lower abdomen or pelvic area; these may be severe.
- Passage of the fetus and other products of conception.

First Aid Measures
Aims: Reassure and comfort the casualty, and arrange for urgent transportation to hospital.
- Reassure the casualty and keep her warm. Lay her down with head and shoulders raised and knees slightly bent, supported by a cushion or blanket.
- Check her pulse and breathing rate.
- Place a sanitary pad or clean towel over her vagina.
- Keep material products of conception for medical inspection.

- If bleeding is continuous and severe, minimize shock by applying treatment for shock. If the woman is lying on a bed, raise the foot for 30–45 cm (12"–18").
- Arrange urgent transportation to hospital.

> **Note:**
> It may not be possible to follow the above procedure, where there are fractures to the upper or lower body; when the casualty is lying in a confined space or if the bent limbs cannot be used as props. In such cases, the recovery position can be maintained by laying a rolled blanket down the front of body. This method can also be used to transport a casualty on a stretcher in the recovery position.

REVIEW QUESTIONS

LONG ESSAYS

1. Classify hemorrhage. Explain the general management for hemorrhage.
2. Define hemorrhage. Describe about severe external bleeding.
3. List the signs and symptoms of hemorrhage and mention the various methods for controlling blood loss.

SHORT ESSAYS

1. Management of bleeding from scalp wound.
2. Internal bleeding and its management.
3. First aid measures for epistaxis.
4. Explain direct pressure.
5. First aid management for ear bleeding.

3.3: SHOCK

Chapter Outline

- Definition
- Causes
- Stages of Shock
- Classification of Shock
- Signs and Symptoms
- First Aid Management

INTRODUCTION

Shock is a life-threatening condition that requires immediate treatment, it can also lead to permanent organ damage. Shock occurs due to sudden drop of blood flow in the body, which arise when cells and organs do not get enough oxygen and nutrients to function properly. Certain elements are necessary for appropriate blood flow to the tissues and cells which includes: an adequate heart pump, an efficient vasculature or circulatory system, and enough blood volume. Blood flow to the tissues is threatened or compromized when one or more element is disturbed.

DEFINITION

- Shock is defined as a condition in which systemic blood pressure is inadequate to deliver oxygen and nutrients to support vital organs and cellular function (Mikhail, 1999).
- A state of cellular and tissue hypoxia known as shock is caused by either a reduction in oxygen delivery, an increase in oxygen consumption, an insufficient amount of oxygen utilisation, or a combination of these factors.

CAUSES

- Trauma
- Allergic reaction
- Severe infection
- Heat stroke
- Blood or fluid loss
- Poisoning
- Severe burns

STAGES OF SHOCK

Initial stage (1st)	Compensatory stage (2nd)	Progressive stage (3rd)	Irreversible stage (4th)
• Decreased cardiac output • Reduced mean arterial pressure • Increased heart rate • Decreased blood pressure • Thirst, pale, cool, moist skin over the face	• Blood pressure remain normal • Vasoconstriction • Increased heart rate • Increased contractility of the heart • Increased cardiac output • Display of "fight or flight" response • Decreased urine output • Cold and clammy skin	• Impaired perfusion • Anaerobic metabolism • Cellular perfusion • Vasoconstriction	• Severe multiple organ damage • Patient does not respond to treatment • Blood pressure continue to remain low • Complete renal and liver failure • Death is imminent

CLASSIFICATION OF SHOCK

1. **Hypovolemic shock:** Shock that occurs due to decreased intravascular volume resulting from fluid loss. It is characterized by rapid, irregular and thread pulse with urine output less than 20 mL/hr.
   a. *Hemorrhagic shock:* Shock occurs due to severe bleeding.
   b. *Traumatic shock:* Shock occurs due to severe injury or wound cause by external force.
   c. *Surgical shock:* Shock that occurs during surgical procedures such as internal hemorrhage, external hemorrhage.
   d. *Burn shock:* Shock that occurs due to decrease cerebral blood flow from burns.
   e. *Dehydration shock:* Shock that occurs due to decrease water content in the body.
2. **Cardiogenic shock:** Shock that result from impairment or failure of the myocardium or inability of the heart to pump blood causing inadequate supply of oxygen to the heart and tissues. It is characterized by angina pain, dysrhythmia and hemodynamic instability.
   a. *Shock due to arrhythmia:* This leads to reduced cardiac output.

b. *Shock due to ischemia:* Results in depressed activity of myocardium.
c. *Shock due to heart failure:* Congestive cardiac disease.
3. **Circulatory or distributive shock:** Shock occurs when there is impaired distribution of blood flow and excessive vasodilation. Types of circulatory or distributive shock includes:
   a. *Septic shock:* Shock occurs due to severe infection characterized by rapid heart rate, warm, pink extremities and widening pulse pressure.
   b. *Anaphylactic shock:* Shock is caused by severe allergic reaction. It is manifested by feeling warm, abdominal pain, diarrhea, flushing, pruritus, urticarial.
   c. *Neurogenic shock:* Shock is cause due to vasodilation that occurs as a result of loss of sympathetic tone. It is manifested by bradycardia, hypotension, hypothermia, dry warm skin.
4. **Obstructive shock**
   a. *Shock due to myocardial tumor*
   b. *Shock due to cardiac tamponade*
   c. *Shock due to pulmonary vascular obstruction:* This occurs due to lungs embolism.

SIGNS AND SYMPTOMS

Signs and symptoms may vary according to the type of shock. Common signs and symptoms includes:
- Pale skin
- Increase pulse rate
- Cool and clammy skin
- Rapid breathing
- Anxious and agitation
- Fatigue
- Dizziness or fainting
- Dilated pupils
- Bluish lips or fingernails

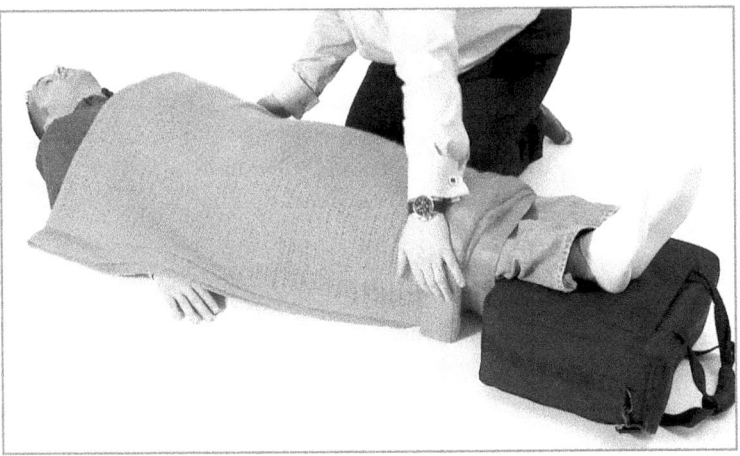

Fig. 3.3.1: Leg and feet elevation.

FIRST AID MANAGEMENT

- If the casualty is conscious, lay him/her down with legs and feet slightly raised and supported **(Fig. 3.3.1)**.
- Position of his/her head on the side to allow saliva to drain from the mouth.
- Loosen any constricting clothing around neck, chest and waist to assist circulation and breathing.
- Do not give the casualty anything by mouth.
- If the casualty becomes unconscious, open his/her airway and check breathing. Complete the CAB of resuscitation, if required and place him/her in the recovery position.
- Follow DRSABCD—Danger, Response, Send, Airway, Breathing, CPR, Defibrillation.
- In case of anaphylactic shock administer epinephrine auto injector if available.
- If casualty is bleeding severely, put pressure over the bleeding area using cloth or sheet.
- Turn the person onto a side to avoid choking if they vomit or start bleeding from the mouth and there is no indication of a spinal injury.
- Arrange urgent transportation to hospital. Transport as a stretcher case maintaining the treatment position.

REVIEW QUESTIONS

LONG ESSAYS

1. Define shock. Explain first aid management of shock.
2. List the classification of shock with explanation.
3. Describe the causes and stage of shock.

SHORT ESSAYS

1. Hypovolemic shock.
2. Cardiogenic shock.
3. Signs and symptoms of shock.
4. Distributive shock.
5. Anaphylactic shock.

Musculoskeletal Injuries 4

4.1: FRACTURE, MUSCLE INJURIES AND DISLOCATION

CHAPTER OUTLINE

- Fracture
- First Aid Measure for Special Cases of Fracture
- First Aid Injuries to Joints and Muscles
- Dislocation

INTRODUCTION

A bone fracture is a medical condition that requires immediate attention; it can occur as a result of a fall, a traffic accident, or bone stress. Adults are prone to radial, femoral, ankle, humerus, and metacarpal fractures. Humerus, ulna, radius, tibia, and fibula fractures are common in children.

FRACTURE

A break or cracked in the bone is known as fracture.

Causes of Fracture

- ❖ **Direct force:** When the bone breaks at the place where force is applied, e.g., a severe blow or crushed by a wheel.
- ❖ **Indirect force:** When a bone breaks at another place and not where the force was applied, the force being transmitted through other bones without injuring them, e.g., a fall on the outstretched hand may result in a fractured clavicle.
- ❖ **Muscle action:** The patella may be broken by a sudden jerk of the knee.
- ❖ **Diseased bone or the brittle bones** of old age breaks easily with very little force.

Types of Fractures

1. **Simple or closed:** When there is no open wound communicating with the fracture.
2. **Compound or open:** When there is a wound communicating with the fracture. In such cases, germs can penetrate to the site of the fracture.
3. **Complicated:** When in connection with the fracture, there is injury to some important internal parts, e.g., lung, brain, spinal cord, or a nerve or large blood vessel. A complicated fracture may be either simple or compound.
4. **Communicated fracture:** The bone is broken into several pieces.
5. **Impacted fracture:** The broken ends are driven into one another.
6. **Depressed fracture:** A fracture of the skull when a broken part is driven inwards.
7. **Green stick fracture:** This fracture occurs in children, when bone is cracked and bent without breaking completely across. A fracture dislocation may occur when the broken bone is close to a joint.

Signs and Symptoms of Fractures

- Pain and tenderness at the site.
- **Loss of power:** The injured part cannot be moved normally.
- Swelling.
- Discoloration may appear soon after the injury or after few days.
- Deformity, normal shape is altered or the limb is shortened.
- Irregularity if the broken bone is close under the skin or protruding.
- Unnatural movement and crepitus (grating sound), only a doctor may examine for these signs.
- Shock.
- The snap of bone may have been heard or felt.

First Aid Treatment of Fractures

Aims

- To prevent further damage, e.g., a simple fracture becoming compound or complicated.
- To prevent pain.
- To make the patient as comfortable as possible until proper treatment is available.
- To prevent shock becoming worse.

Rules

- Do not move the patient or limb unless in danger.
- Be steady and support the injured part at once, and prevent movement.
- Reassure the patient and send for medical aid if possible.
- Stop hemorrhage if any, and cover wounds with dry dressing. Do not remove clothing unnecessarily.
- Counteract shock by handling gently, keeping warm, reassuring and giving sweet fluids. If an anesthetic is likely to be given soon, give nothing by mouth.
- Immobilize the injured part. A broken arm may be tied to the body or a broken leg to the other unaffected leg or splints may be used.
- Never do more than is necessary.
- Arrange for suitable transport to hospital. A firm stretcher is needed, or a plank or door if there is fracture of a leg or the spine.

First Aid Measures for Special Cases of Fracture

Fracture of the Skull

The brain may be injured and unconsciousness develops. There may be bleeding from ear or nose.

- After any head injury, the patient should be carefully watched and taken to a doctor.
- The patient should be kept quiet, lying with the head turned to one side.
- If there is a wound, a dressing should be applied.
- Keep the head still while transporting the patient to hospital.

Fracture of the Spine

There is danger of paralysis due to injury of the spinal cord.

- Warn the patient to be still.
- Treat for shock until sufficient help is available to lift the patient carefully onto a stretcher and transport to hospital.
- Tie the patient's legs together with padding between the ankles, knees and thighs.
- At least four people are needed to lift him/her onto the stretcher. It is important not to bend or twist the spine when moving the patient.
- The best position is which to transport him/her is lying on back with small pillows or pads under the hollow of the neck and the small of the back. These should first be placed in position on the stretcher

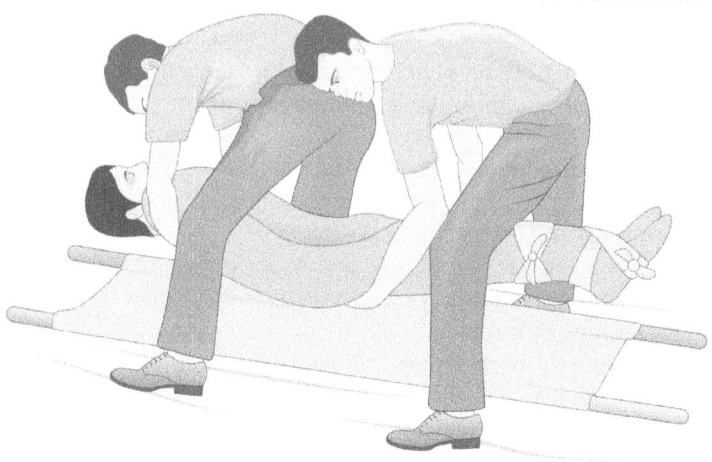

Fig. 4.1.1: Lifting of spinal injury patient.

(**Fig. 4.1.1**). A door or board may be used as a stretcher, and the patient is tied firm to it to prevent movement during transport.

Fracture of the Ribs

The special danger is that the broken ribs may be driven inwards causing a complicated fracture. There will be great pain on breathing and blood may be coughed up. First aid measures should be done by providing support to the patient in the most comfortable position usually or two broad bandages overlapping may be applied to the chest and tied tightly just after the patient has breathed out, and the arm may be supported in a sling.

Fracture of Clavicle

Clavicle fracture is often caused by indirect force, such as fall on the outstretched hand. The arm of injured side should be supported. Pad well between the upper arm and the side of the chest. Tie the arm to the chest with a broad bandage, then apply a St John sling (**Fig. 4.1.2**).

Fractures of the Upper Limb

The humerus may be fractured close to the shoulder, in the middle of the shaft or near the elbow joint. A Colles' fracture is common, the lower end of the radius is being broken. Fractures of the metacarpals may cause severe bleeding into the palm of the hand. The bandaging of the palm is shown in **Figure 4.1.3**.

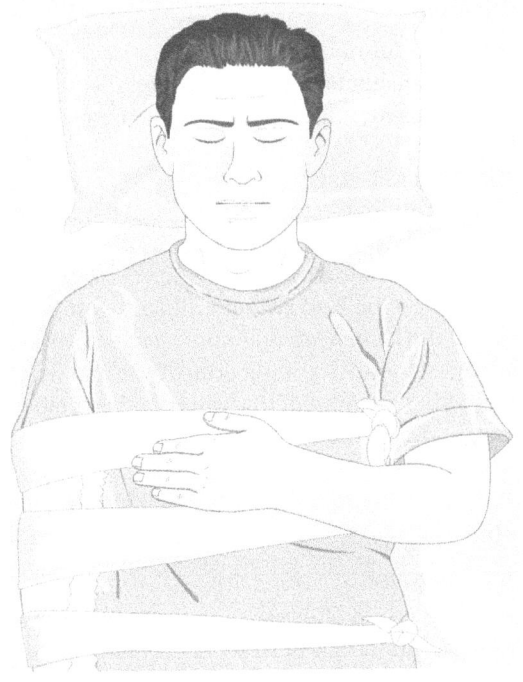

Fig. 4.1.2: Bandaging fractured arm with triangular bandage.

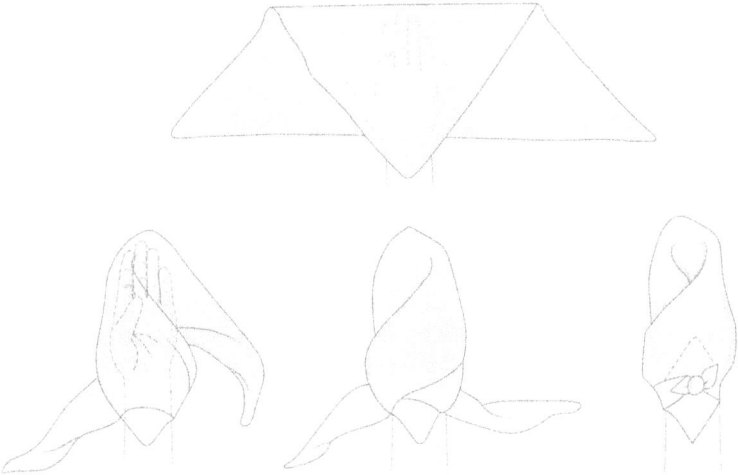

Fig. 4.1.3: Palm bandaging with triangular bandage.

First Aid Measures

- The limb must be immobilized.
- If the elbow can be bent without increasing the pain, flex the arm against the chest with fingers touching the opposite shoulder.
- Put some padding between the limb and the chest and fix the hand with a collar and cuff sling.
- Bind the arm firmly to the chest by two broad bandages, one round the upper arm near to the shoulder, and the other near to the elbow, tying off on the opposite side of the body.
- If the elbow cannot be bent without difficulty or increasing pain, tie the limb to the trunk with padding between by means of three broad bandages, round the upper arm, elbow and wrist, or a splint may be applied to the front of the arm from just below the armpit to the wrist, and tied with broad bandages above and below the fracture and round the wrist.
- Transport the patient in sitting or lying position whichever is more comfortable.

Fracture of the Forearm

The arm-to-body method of fixing can be used as above, but if this causes discomfort, splints may be used. The forearm should be placed across the chest with thumb uppermost, and palm of the hand towards the body. Well-padded splints should be applied to front and back of the forearm from the elbow to the fingers. Fix the splints by means of two narrow bandages; one applied above the fracture, the other as a figure-of-eight round the hand and wrist. Support the arm in a large arm sling with fingers slightly higher than the elbow (**Fig. 4.1.4**). Watch the fingers for signs of interference with circulation in which case, loosen the bandages slightly.

Fracture of the Pelvis

The patient will be unable to stand; pelvic organs, especially bladder or urethra, may be injured, and the patient may have desire to pass urine, but have difficulty in doing so. He/she should be told not to try. A firm binder, towel or two broad bandages overlapping are applied round the pelvis tying on sound side. Ankles and knees together lift carefully onto the stretcher supporting the pelvis well.

Fracture of the Femur

Fracture of the neck of the femur is common in elderly people or the fracture may be anywhere in the shaft. There will be a good deal of

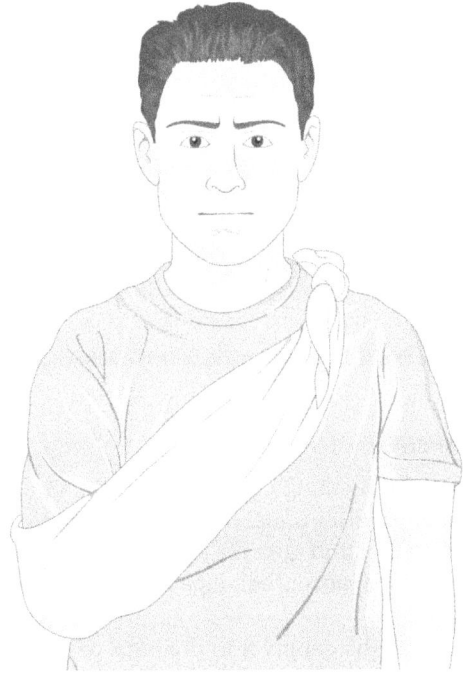

Fig. 4.1.4: Large arm sling with triangular bandage.

shock. Shortening of the leg is often noticed, and the foot has it on its outer side. First aid measures for fracture of femur should be done as follows:

- Pad between the legs, and bring the good leg alongside the injured one.
- Tie together the knees, ankles, hips, above and below the site of fracture.
- If there is a long or difficult journey to hospital, two well-padded splints should be used; one between the legs and a long one on the outer side of the body extending from the armpit to the foot.
- Secure with bandages round the chest, pelvis, knees, above and below the fracture, lower legs and a figure-of-eight around both ankles and feet.

Fracture of the Lower Leg

Treat same as for fracture of the femur, omitting the long splint. Positioning for leg fracture is shown in **Figure 4.1.5**.

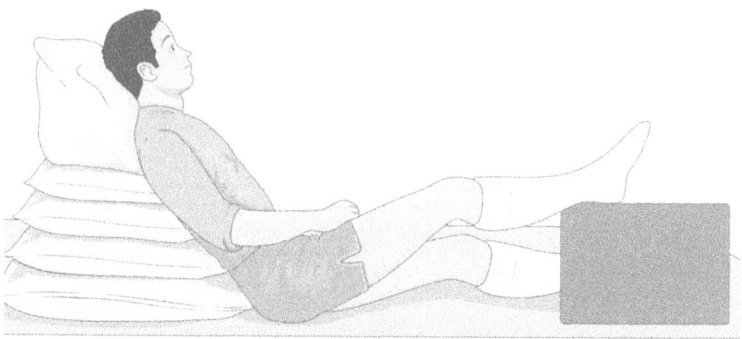

Fig. 4.1.5: Positioning for leg fracture.

Fracture of the Patella

Support the patient in sitting position. Raise the injured leg gently, and place the uninjured leg under it for support (crossed leg method). Tie the ankles together and raise the legs on a box. The legs may also be tied together with a narrow bandage above and below the knee in a figure-of-eight.

If a splint is available, apply it to the back of the limb. It should reach from the buttock to beyond the heel. Pad under the ankle and secure the splint to the limb by bandages round the thigh, ankle, and figure-of-eight above and below the knee.

FIRST AID INJURIES TO JOINTS AND MUSCLES

Strain

A strain is the overstretching of a muscle due to a sudden effort or twisting of the part. Strain is an injury to a muscle or a tendon leading to tearing of muscle fibers as shown in **Figure 4.1.6**.

Sign and Symptoms

There is sudden sharp pain in the muscle, and movement causes more pain. There may be swelling.

Treatment
- Rest and support patient in the most comfortable position.
- Support the injured part.
- Use slings, bandages or adhesive plaster.

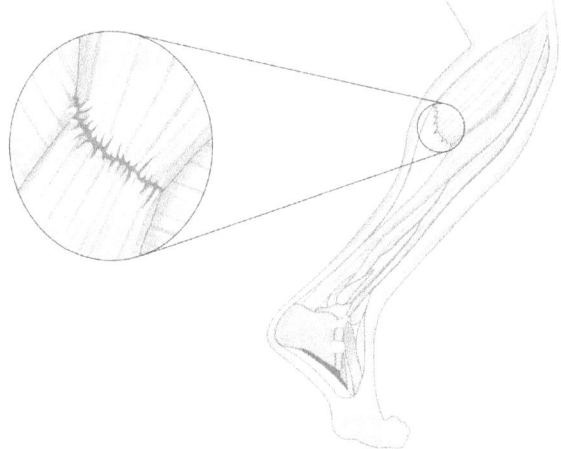

Fig. 4.1.6: Calf muscle strain.

Sprain

A sprain is a joint injury with tearing of ligaments caused by sudden twisting of the joint. The ankle is the most common joint to be sprained **(Fig. 4.1.7)**, the external ligament being torn due to falling with the foot turned inwards. There will be severe pain, and some joints become very swollen. The tear may be a complete tear or tear of part of the ligament.

Signs and Symptoms

- Severe pain at the time of injury. The pain becomes less later, but as the bruise increases, the pain also increases and is maximum after about 4 hours.
- Swelling of the joint.
- Discoloration around the joint (bruising) due to the collection of blood.
- Loss of movement at the joint. Unnatural movement, creaking and deformity are absent; this excludes a fracture.

Treatment

- Apply a firm bandage before swelling occurs, if possible.
- Get the patient or a helper to hold the foot up at right angles to the leg.

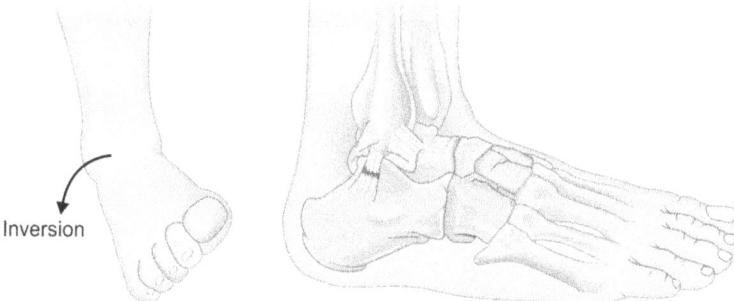

Fig. 4.1.7: Ankle sprain.

- Place a pad of cotton wool or cloth on the outer side, then start the bandage first round the lower part of the leg just above the ankle.
- Then under the heel, and up on the outer side to give support, and again covering the first turn.
- Repeat the turns alternately, gradually working towards the point of the heel.
- Wet the bandage with cold water and keep it wet. This will tighten the bandage and help prevent swelling.
- Encourage the patient to walk on the ankle or at least to keep moving the joint in all those directions which do not cause acute pain.
- The patient should be taken to a doctor. If one is doubtful about whether it is a sprain or a fracture, treat it as a fracture.

Bruise

A bruise is a soft tissue injury **(Fig. 4.1.8)** that involves the skin and nearby tissues as a result of a blow or other force that breaks a blood vessel near the body's surface. Bruising can occur as a result of a sprain or strain.

Signs and Symptoms
- Discoloration of skin.
- Pain during the first few days.
- Swelling.

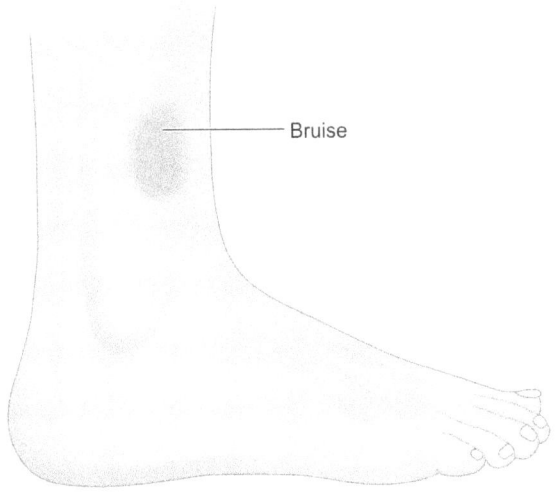

Fig. 4.1.8: Bruise.

Treatment

- Place the patient in comfortable position.
- Apply rest, ice, compression, elevation.
- If there is visible bruising use a compression bandage.

Dislocation

A dislocation is a displacement of the bones, which form a joint **(Fig. 4.1.9)**. Joints most commonly dislocated are the shoulder (in adults), elbow (in children), lower jaw, thumb and fingers. There will be severe pain in the joint, which feels useless and fixed. There will be some deformity (difference in shape when compared with the other limb) and swelling occurs later.

Signs and Symptoms

- Severe pain at or near the joint.
- Loss of normal joint movements.
- Deformity when compared with the other joint.
- Swelling caused by the collection of blood.

Treatment

- Do not try to put the bone back in place.
- Support the limb in the position most comfortable for the patient.

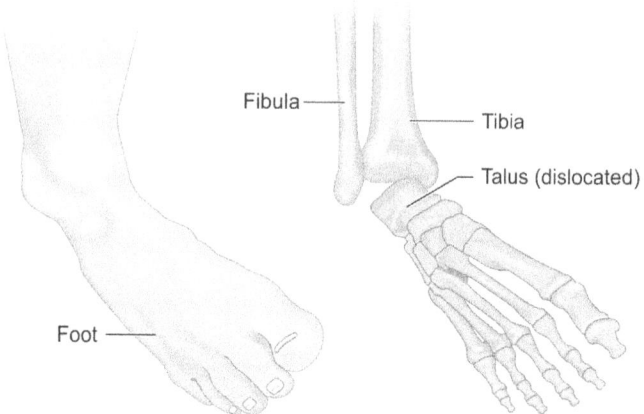

Fig. 4.1.9: Dislocated ankle.

- Immobilize the part as in treating a fracture.
- Take the patient to a doctor quickly.

REVIEW QUESTIONS

LONG ESSAYS

1. Describe fracture and explain the first aid treatment of fracture in details.
2. Discuss first aid measures for special cases of fracture.
3. Explain in detail regarding sprain and strain.

SHORT ESSAYS

1. Define fracture. Explain the types of fracture.
2. Bruise and its first aid management.
3. Dislocation.
4. First aid measures for fracture of upper limbs.
5. Fracture of spine.

4.2: INJURIES: HEAD, SPINAL CORD AND OTHERS

CHAPTER OUTLINE

- Head Injuries
- Concussion
- Spinal Cord Injury
- Others: Injury to an Extremity, Lower Jaw Injury, Dental Injury

INTRODUCTION

Children, adolescents, and adults frequently sustain minor head injuries and concussions. Many different signs and symptoms of a concussion include dizziness or nausea after recovery, forgetfulness of any events that happened during or immediately before the injury, and a mild, generalized headache. Some of these coexist with different illnesses. In most head injuries, loss of consciousness is rare, and if it persists for more than 30 seconds, it might be a sign of a more serious internal head injury. Although there is conflicting evidence regarding first aid professionals' ability to recognize a spinal injury, they should have a high index of suspicion based on the events that have taken place and treat the patient as though a spinal injury were present.

HEAD INJURIES

An injury that occurs to the scalp, skull, brain, tissues and blood vessels associated with the head.

- In any case of head trauma, if unconsciousness lasts for more than a minute, the victim needs urgent observation and care.
- Victim who have suffered a minor closed head injury and have experienced a 1-minute loss of consciousness should be examined and monitored by a medical professional.
- Minor closed head injury victims who do not lose consciousness can be observed at home under the care of a qualified caregiver.
- While evaluating the victim, first aider must pay attention to the airway and breathing.

Signs and Symptoms of Head Injuries

- Severe pain in the head.
- Change in level of consciousness.

- Bleeding from scalp.
- Difficulty in breathing and vision.
- Nausea and vomiting
- Either slow or fast pulse.
- Bruising of the head, especially around the eyes, ears/nose.

First Aid Measures

- Apply pressure bandage **(Fig. 4.2.1)**, if bleeding is present.
- Assess the airway, breathing and circulation.
- Observe carefully for pulse, breathing, color of skin, lips and nails.
- Treat for shock.
- Transport the patient to nearby hospital in recovery position.

Concussion

A concussion is a traumatic injury to the brain that is caused by a blow to the head or a violent shaking of the head.

Signs and Symptoms of Head Injury

- Feeling of pressure in the head.
- Nausea or vomiting.
- Dizziness or blurry vision may be present.
- Sensitivity to light and noise.
- Confusion or disorientation.

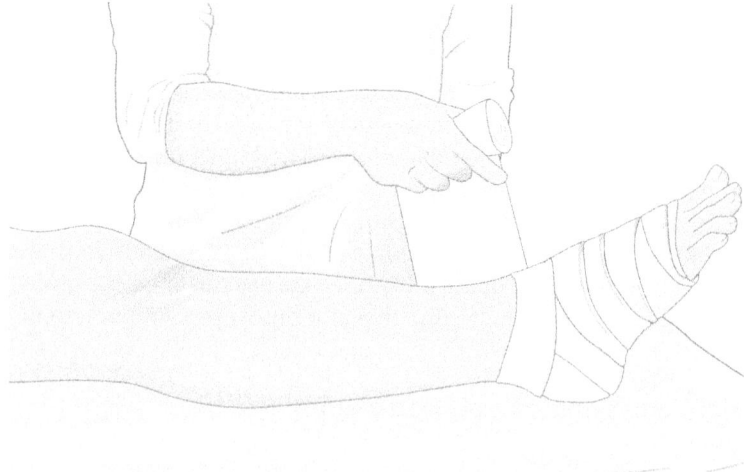

Fig. 4.2.1: Applying pressure bandage on the limb.

First Aid Measures
- The victim needs to take physical and mental rest until his/her condition improves.
- The three R's steps should be followed—**R**ecognize, **R**eport and **R**ecover.
- Apply a cold compressed to the injury to reduce swelling.
- There is no proper cure for concussion, any person who sustain a concussion should only be evaluated and treat by healthcare professionals.
- A person with concussion should avoid doing any physical activities until they recover.

SPINAL INJURY

Spinal cord injury is an injury that results from damage to the spinal column's vertebrae, ligaments, discs, or spinal cord itself. A sudden, traumatic blow to the spine that fractures, dislocates, crushes, or compresses one or more of your vertebrae can result in a traumatic spinal cord injury.

It is essential for first responders to assume that any head injury may be associated with spinal injury as they cannot definitively determine whether a victim has a spinal injury, they should be on the lookout for it if they notice any of the following risk factors:
- 65 years old or older.
- Victims of motor vehicle crash.
- Falls form a height greater than standing height.
- Tingling sensation in the extremities.
- Pain or tenderness in the neck or back.
- Evidence of head or neck trauma in children below 3 years of age.
- Disoriented.

Signs and Symptoms for Damage Spinal Cord
- Pain at the area of injury or neck.
- Loss of control on the limb.
- Casualty may complain that limbs feel stiff, heavy or clumsy.
- Loss of bowel and bladder control.
- Breathing difficulties.

First Aid Measures
The aim is to prevent further injury, ensure airway is clear, transportation of casualty to the nearby hospital.
- If spinal injury is suspected, the first aider must immobilize the casualty.

SECTION 2: First Aid Management

- ❖ Keep the casualty's head in a neutral position and place rolled-up blankets, towels, or articles of clothing on either side of the casualty's head and neck as shown in **Figure 4.2.2A**.
- ❖ Advise the casualty not to move.
- ❖ Put your knees behind the casualty head. With your hands covering the casualty ears, firmly grasp the sides of his or her head. The casualty should still be able to hear you if you do not completely cover their ears. In the neutral head position, where the head, neck, and spine are in alignment, keep your head steady and support it **(Fig. 4.2.2B)**. This is the least dangerous head position for a victim with a suspected spinal injury.

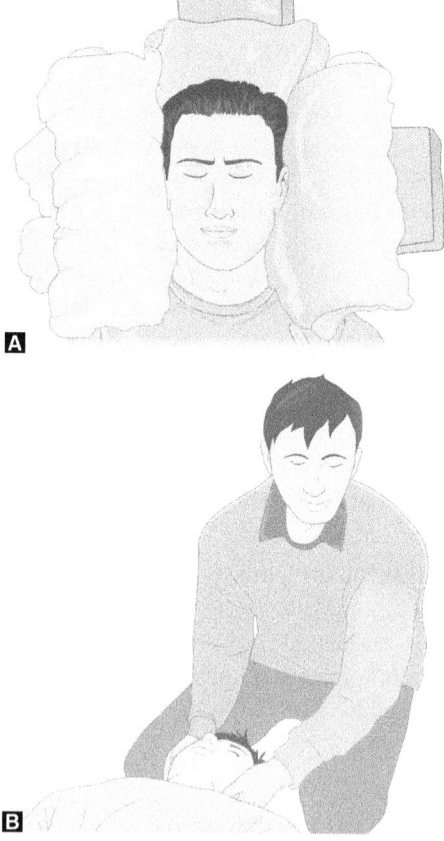

Figs. 4.2.2A and B: (A) Placing roll up towels on both sides of the casualty head and neck; (B) Positioning of patient head in neutral position.

- No matter how long it takes, keep holding the casualty's head in a neutral position until emergency medical services arrive.
- Get help to monitor and record vital signs, such as the responsiveness level, pulse, and breathing.
- Continue further assessment to identify any other injury in the body.
- Bandage the legs to immobilize them if the casualty is moving his or her leg due to pain. This will come in handy when using the log-roll technique while transporting. The log-roll technique can be applied to either conscious or unconscious casualties.
- If an unconscious casualty's airway is blocked and the jaw thrust technique is ineffective, use the log-roll technique.

Log-roll technique (Figs. 4.2.3A and B): If you need to turn a casualty with a spinal injury, use this technique. The move can be completed with three people instead of five. While you support the casualty's head and neck, instruct your helpers to gently straighten the limbs. Then, while ensuring that everyone is working together, roll the casualty. Maintain a straight line between the casualty's head, trunk, and toes at all times. Support the casualty's neck and head before lowering them onto a hard plank or hard stretcher and transporting them to an ambulance.

OTHERS

1. **Injury to an extremity:** Injury to an extremity can be painful but it is not life-threatening. Depending on the nature of the injury it be associated with bleeding, fracture, immobility. The goal is to preserve the extremity and to limit pain, bleeding, and transportation to nearby medical facilities.
   Signs and symptoms
   - Pain at the injured area or surrounding area.
   - Bleeding.
   - Swelling and discoloration.
   - Loss of normal shape.
   - Immobility.
   - Bone irregularity.

   First aid measures
   - Priority is to immobile the injured part.

SECTION 2: First Aid Management

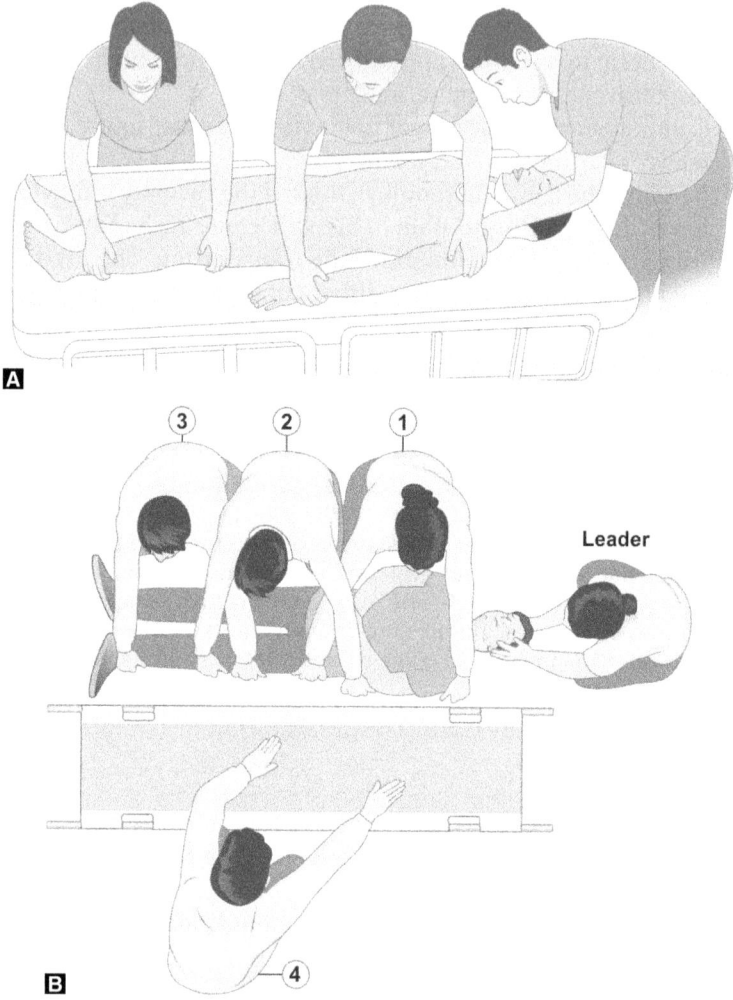

Figs. 4.2.3A and B: Log-roll technique.

- If it is sprain or soft tissue injury, apply cold therapy for not more than 20 minutes.
- Provide support to the injured area.
- Expose the site of injury.
- Treat the wounds and apply bandages or splint as required. Refer chapter 3.1 for different types of wound with first aid measures.

2. **Lower jaw injury:** Any injury to the jaw is caused due to an accidents, it can be broken or dislocated.
   First aid measures
   - Instruct the patient not to speak and eat anything by mouth.
   - Assess for airway and make sure the tongue does not fall back. Removes dentures if present.
   - Place your hand or the palm of the patient's hand on the chin, gently press the lower jaw up against the upper jaw (which serves as a splint), and lean forward.
   - Put a small bandage underneath the chin. Cross the other end over the ear while carrying one end up and over the top of the head. Carry the shorter end across the front of the forehead and the longer end around the back of the head in the opposite direction. Tie the other end just above the ear **(Fig. 4.2.4)**.
   - If the victim exhibits vomiting symptoms, remove the bandage and re-tie it when the vomiting stops.
   - Transport him to hospital as early as possible.
3. **Dental injury:** Physical injury to the teeth, gums, alveolar bone (the bone that holds the tooth sockets), or soft tissue of the mouth, including the lips and tongue, is referred to as dental trauma. It is common among children.

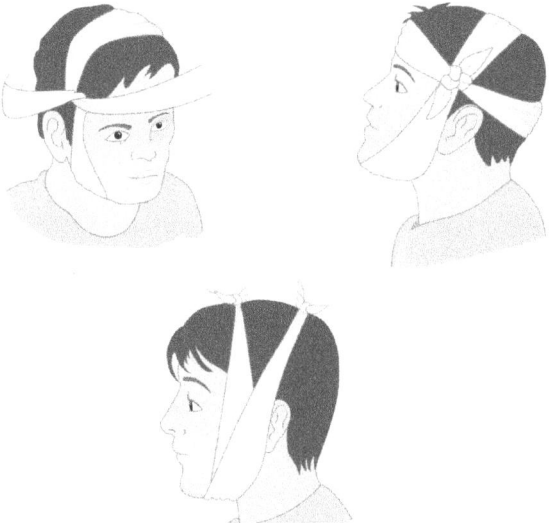

Fig. 4.2.4: Bandaging lower jaw.

First aid measures

The first aider must not avulsed the teeth instead, they should store it in milk (if available) or water and transported with the injured casualty to a dentist or hospital.

- Clean the wound with water.
- In case of bleeding, stop the bleeding by applying pressure with clean gauze or cotton.
- Handle the tooth by the crown (top), not the root. Do not handle the part below the gum line.
- Place the tooth in milk, if milk is not available use water.

REVIEW QUESTIONS

LONG ESSAYS

1. Describe spinal injury and its first aid measures.
2. Explain head injuries in detail.
3. Elaborate the different types of injuries and explain concussion in details.

SHORT ESSAYS

1. Lower jaw injury.
2. Injury to the extremities.
3. Dental injury.
4. Define spinal injury and list its signs and symptoms.
5. Explain log-roll technique.

4.3: BANDAGES AND DRESSINGS

CHAPTER OUTLINE

- Bandages
- Slings
- Splints

INTRODUCTION

Bandages and dressings are used to provide support to restrict the movement of a body part. In some cases both dressing and bandages are used together, where the dressing is applied directly to the wound, and a bandage is used to keep it in place. Dressing is used for covering a break in skin to help control the bleeding.

BANDAGES

Bandages are soft, absorbent gauze or other material that is applied to a limb or other part of the body.

Purpose of Bandages

Bandage may be used for the following purposes:
- To reduce movement of a joint.
- To retain a splint in position.
- To serve as an improvised tourniquet.
- To keep dressings, poultice or splints in position.
- To give support to a limb or tissues.
- To reduce or prevent swelling.
- To correct deformity.
- To control bleeding.
- To limit movement.

Bandages can be improvised by using any soft clean pieces of cotton cloth such as a handkerchief, a towel or pieces of sheeting. Bandages may be either triangular or long strips. The bandage can be used in three forms:
- In the triangular form.
- In the broad-fold form.
- In the narrow-fold form.

Note:
- Remember that bandaging cannot be learnt from books, but only from constant practice. Illustrations can help, however, for the purpose of reference.
- **Reef knot:** One must always ensure that the knot used in tying a bandage is secured and that there is no danger of its slipping. The knot, which is used in the 'Reef knot' because the more it is tightened, the more secure it becomes. Also it can easily be undone if you want to undo the knot without damaging the bandage.
- Remember that the knot must always be tied away from the injury so that it will not hurt.

Principles of Bandaging (to be Demonstrated)

- It entirely covers the dressing and yet is not cumbersome to the patient.
- It should be firm enough to keep the dressing in place, yet not so tight that it causes discomfort, or impedes circulation (except in case of a bandage applied to stop bleeding).
- It is neat in appearance.

Patterns Used in Bandaging

- **Circular turns:** Circular turns is used to bandage the proximal aspect of a finger or a wrist as shown in **Figure 4.3.1**. Steps includes:
  - Apply the bandage's end to the area of the body that needs bandaging.
  - Encircle the body part several times or as close as possible, with each turn directly covering the previous turn.
  - Over a healthy area, fasten the bandage's end with tape, metal clips, or a safety pin.
- **Simple spiral/spiral turn:** Body parts with relatively uniform circumferences, like the upper arm or upper leg, are bandaged using spiral turns **(Fig. 4.3.2)**. Steps includes:
  - To secure the bandage, make two circular turns.
  - Continue making spiral turns at a 30° angle, overlapping each turn by two-thirds of the bandage's width.
  - Wrap the bandage twice in a circle to finish.
- **Reversed spiral:** Reverse spiral is used on limbs where, owing to varying thickness, a simple spiral bandage would not lie smoothly. It is applied on cylindrical body parts. Steps includes **(Fig. 4.3.3)**:

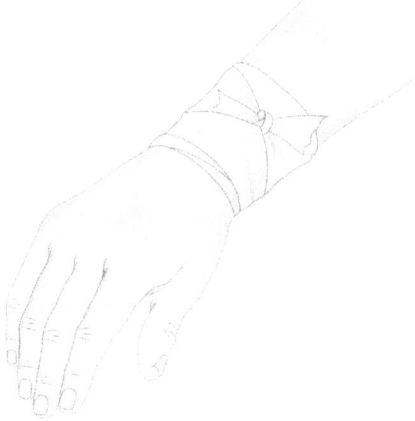

Fig. 4.3.1: Circular bandage.

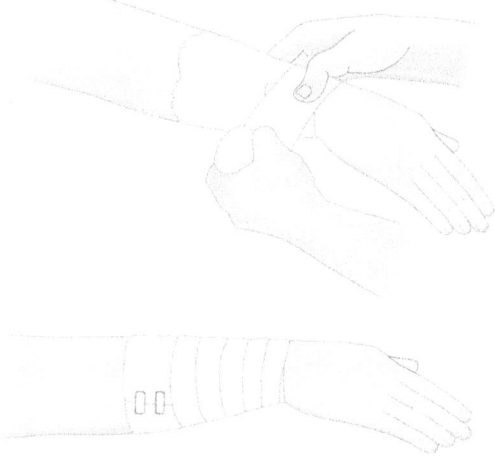

Fig. 4.3.2: Simple spiral bandage.

- Make two circular turns and bring the bandage upwards at about 30° angle.
- On the upper edge of the bandage, place the thumb of the free hand.
- Unroll the bandage around about 15 cm (6 inches) then turn the hand so that the bandage falls over itself.

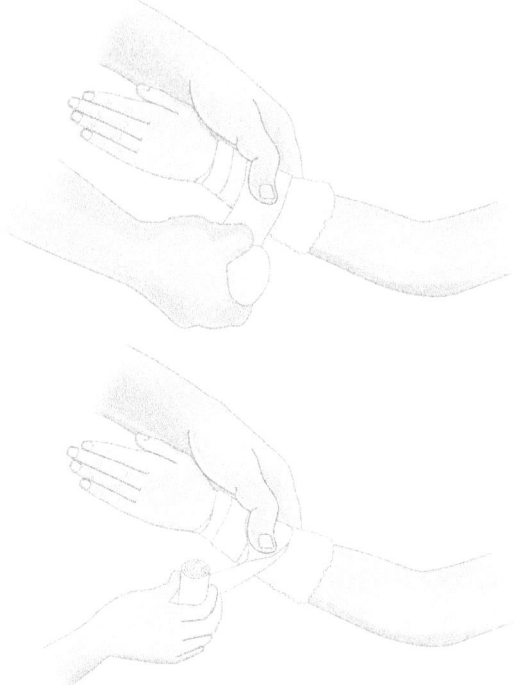

Fig. 4.3.3: Reversed spiral bandage.

- Continue wrapping the bandage around the limb, overlapping each previous turn by two-thirds the width of the bandage, and making each bandage turn at the same position on the limb so that the bandage turns are aligned.
- Secure the bandage with two circular turns.

❖ **Figure-of-eight**: Figure-of-eight **(Fig. 4.3.4)** may be used on limbs instead of the reversed spiral, and for the hand and foot. Following steps shows knee bandage using figure-of-eight:
  - Flex the knee and place the bandage's outer side against the inner side of the knee (medial).
  - Make two straight/circular turns around the kneecap.
  - Turn below and above to cover one-third of the previous turn.
  - Turn below and above the joint until the entire knee is covered.
  - Finish with two circular turns around the thigh to secure the bandage.
  - Use adhesive tape or a safety pin to secure the end.

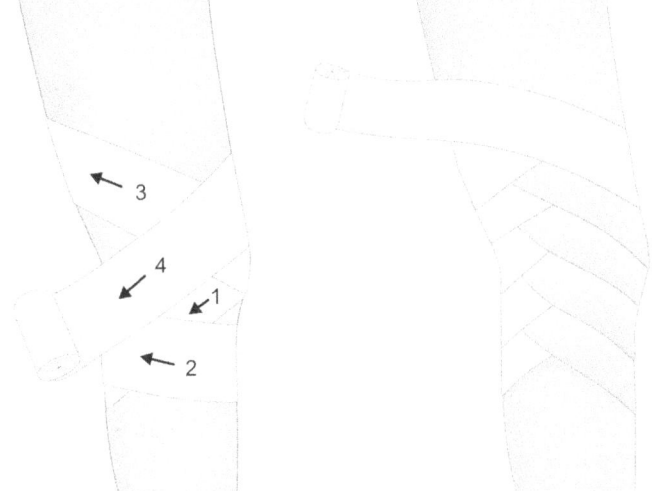

Fig. 4.3.4: Figure of eight.

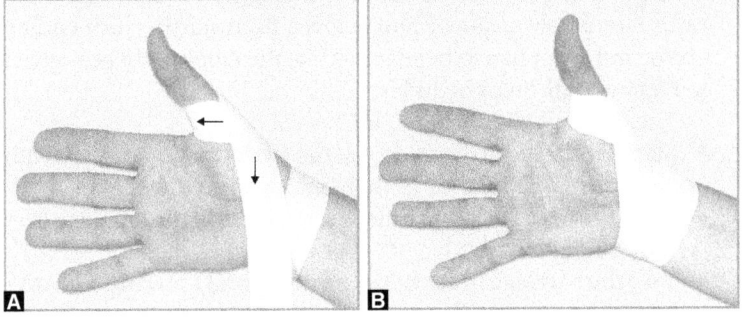

Figs. 4.3.5A and B: Spica of thumb.

❖ **Spica:** The spica is a figure-of-eight in which one turn is significantly larger than the other. It is used for joints that are at right angles to the body, such as the shoulder, groin, and thumb as shown in **Figures 4.3.5A and B**. Steps includes:
  • Bend the elbow at right angles.
  • Place the bandage's outer side on the joint's inner side and make two straight turns carrying the bandage over the elbow tip and around the elbow.
  • Turn a second time to encircle the forearm and upper arm.
  • Ensure that the first turn is one-third the width of the bandage below and above.

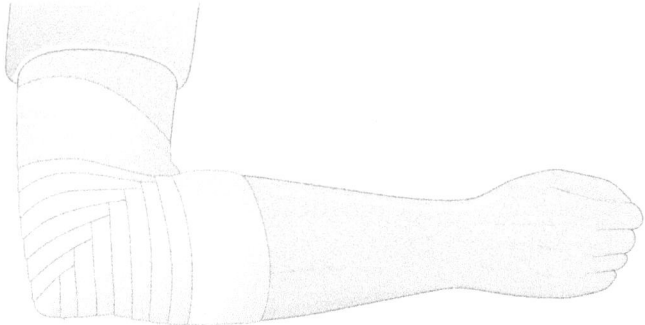

Fig. 4.3.6: Divergent spica of elbow.

- Bandage the remaining one-third of the previous turn until the entire dressing is secured.
- Complete the bandaging by making two circular turns above and securing it with a safety pin or tape.

❖ **Divergent spica:** It is a variation of the figure-of-eight where the turns alternately go above and below a fixed starting turn ending above and is applied to bend joints like the elbow or heel as given in **Figure 4.3.6**. Steps includes:
- The bandage should be 2.5 inches wide.
- Start bandaging at the middle of the elbow or joints and fix with two or three circular turns then, reverse the elbow.
- Once the forearm is fixed, place the middle of the bandage over the point of the elbow.
- Take the bandage from within, forwards and outwards and over lower part of preceding turn.
- Then turn to the inner side again and outwards and over upper part of the first turn and so on.
- Finally, close the elbow with figures of eight.

❖ **Recurrent bandage:** Recurrent bandage is used to cover blunt body parts, tips of fingers or a stump (amputated limb) and are fixed by using circular or spiral turns as shown in **Figure 4.3.7**.
- On the blunt body part, the bandage is repeatedly applied from one side across the top to the opposite side.
- Not only the wound, but the entire length of the blunt body part should be covered in order to effectively fix the recurrent turns.
- Successive turns are made to cover the preceding turn fully or partially.

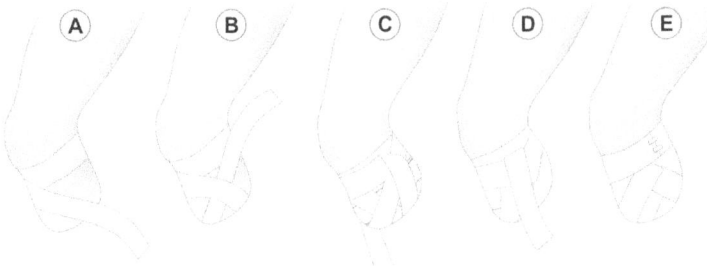

Fig. 4.3.7: Recurrent bandage of stump.

- Special bandages such as capeline for the head, eye, ear and breast bandages.

Types of Bandages

1. Roller bandages
2. Triangular bandages
3. **Special bandages:** tailed bandages.

Roller Bandages

Roller bandages are made of various materials such as gauze, open-woven cotton, calico, flannel, crepe, elastoplast, cotton, rubber (used as a tourniquet) and plaster of Paris. Bandages may be improvised from any available material. Torn into strips of the required length and width, which should be as detailed in **Table 4.3.1**. Roller bandages should be rolled tightly and evenly **(Figs. 4.3.8 to 4.3.10)**, preferably using a bandage roller or the back of a chair. Selvedges are to be avoided.

Table 4.3.1: Roller bandage.

Part of body	Width of bandages	Length of bandages
Finger	½–1 inch	1–3 yard
Hand	1–2 inch	3 yard
Arm	2–2 ½ inch	7–9 yard
Foot	1 ½–3 inch	4 yard
Leg	2–3 inch	9 yard
Body	3–6 inch	10 yard
Head	2 inch	6 yard

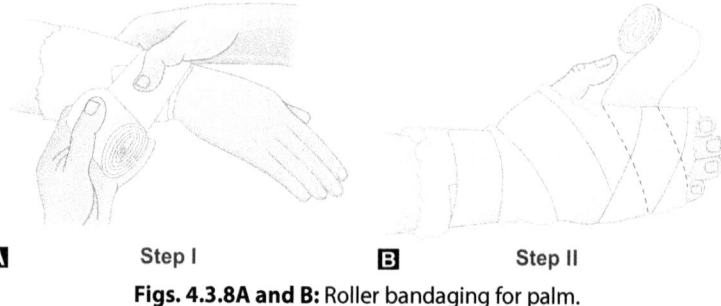

Figs. 4.3.8A and B: Roller bandaging for palm.

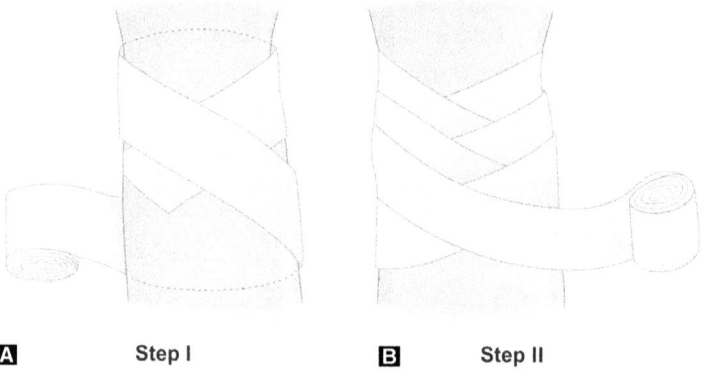

Figs. 4.3.9A and B: Roller bandaging for wrist joint connecting the forearm.

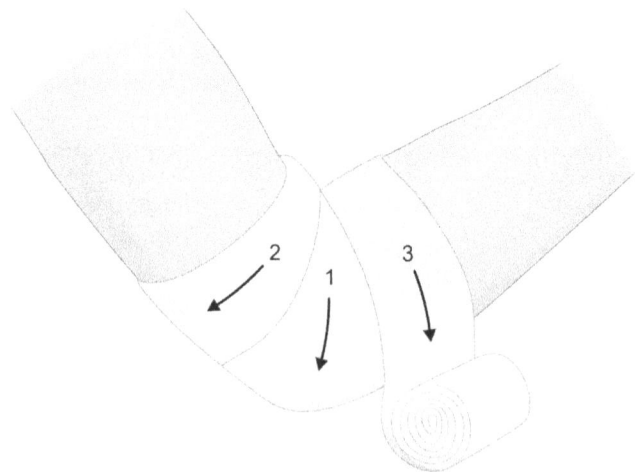

Fig. 4.3.10: Roller bandage for elbow.

Rules for the Application of Roller Bandages

1. Have the patient in a comfortable position, and support the limb to be bandaged in the position in which it is to remain.
2. Stand in front of the patient and the part to be bandaged, except when bandaging the head or back of the neck.
3. Hold the drum of the bandage in the right hand when bandaging a left limb and vice versa.
4. Apply the outer side of the bandage to the part, holding the drum uppermost.
5. Use pads where necessary to avoid pressure or skin surfaces touching, e.g., in axilla.
6. Unroll no more than 2 inches of bandage at a time and maintain even pressure.
7. See that the bandage is neither too tight nor too slack.
8. Bandage from below upwards and within outwards over the front of the limb.
9. Apply each layer of the bandage, so that it covers two thirds of the previous turn.
10. Finish in the front with a safety pin, adhesive plaster or stitching. Do not finish it on top of the wound or on bony prominence.

Triangular Bandages

The triangular bandage is much used in first aid, because it is more suitable than the roller bandage for improvisation. It is also used as a sling to support the arm. It is made of strong cotton cloth.

Steps for Application of Triangular Bandages

- A piece about 36–40 inches or 1 m^2, cut diagonally makes two bandages.
- The edges should be hemmed. The long side is called base and the corner opposite to it is the point.
- The bandage may be applied opened out or it can be folded into a broad or narrow bandage.
- The ankle with triangular bandage is shown in **Figure 4.3.11**.

To Fold a Bandage

- Bring the point down to the center of the base then fold again in the same direction. This makes a 'broad bandage'.
- Fold once again in the same direction to make a 'narrow bandage'.
- When not in use, the triangular bandage should be folded narrow then the two ends are folded to the center, and again in two, making a neat packet.

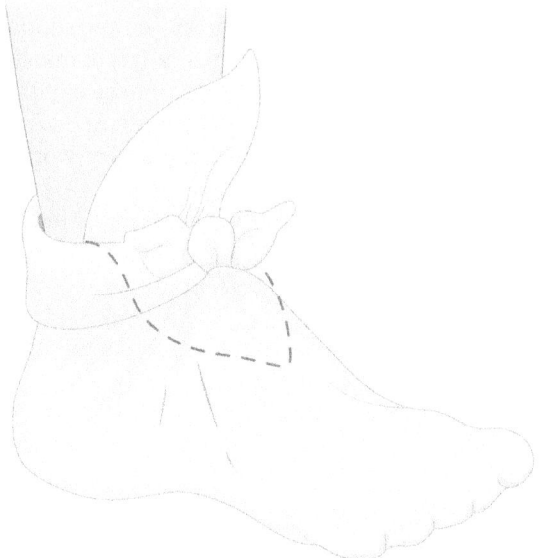

Fig. 4.3.11: Ankle with triangular bandage.

Uses of Triangular Bandage

1. ***Large arm sling:*** Large arm sling is used for support in most cases of injury to the arm, hand or fingers **(Fig. 4.3.17)**.
   Method:
   - Place the open bandage on the chest so that one end is long enough to pass round the neck to the injured side, and the point of the triangle passes behind the elbow.
   - Bend the arm so that the hand is higher than the elbow.
   - Bring the lower end of the bandage up to tie in front of the injured side.
   - Bring the point forward, turn it in, if necessary, and pin neatly in front.
2. ***Hand bandage (Fig. 4.3.12A):*** Hand bandage is used for retaining hand dressings.
   Method:
   - Place the hand on the open bandage with fingers toward the point.
   - Bring the point down over the hand above the wrist.

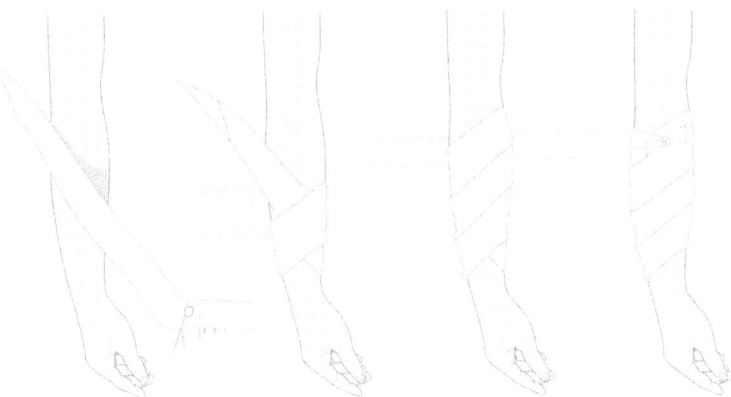

Fig. 4.3.12A: Triangular hand bandage.

- Cross the ends round the wrist (two or three times as necessary).
- Tie the ends of the bandage over the wrist.
- Pin the point down over the knot.

Note:
Make sure that the knot over the wrist is not too tight to obstruct the pulse

3. **Foot bandage (Fig. 4.3.12B):** Foot bandage is used to retain dressings on the foot.
   Method:
   - Place the foot on an open bandage, toes towards the point.
   - Bring the point up to the ankle.
   - Cross the ends round the ankle and tie the ends in front of the ankle.
   - Pin the point down over the knot.
4. **Joint bandaging (Fig. 4.3.12C):** The method of using the open triangular bandage is essentially the same for every joint. It is used to retain dressings, where a roller bandage would be bulky and uncomfortable.
   Method:
   - Apply the triangular bandage to the part, pointing uppermost, and adjust the size by folding up the base as necessary.
   - Take the ends in each hand and carry them round behind the part. Cross them, thus changing hands at the back.

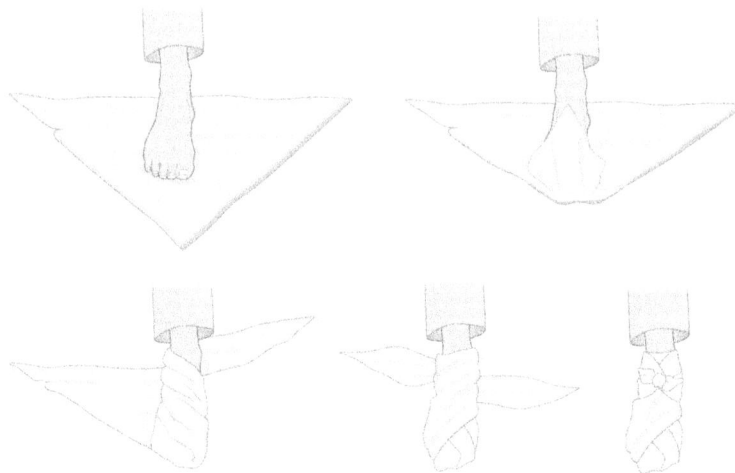

Fig. 4.3.12B: Triangular foot bandage.

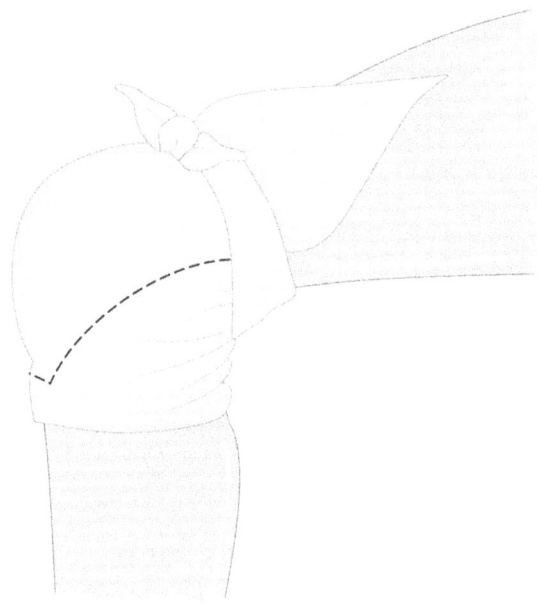

Fig. 4.3.12C: Triangular joint bandage.

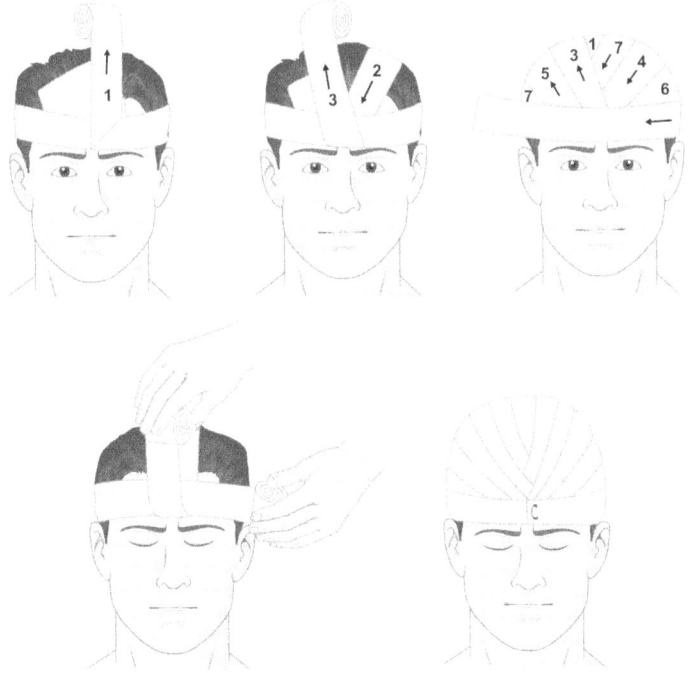

Fig. 4.3.12D: Triangular scalp/capeline bandage.

- Bring the ends round to the front and tie them.
- Pin down the point of the bandage.
5. ***Scalp/capeline bandage (Fig. 4.3.12D):*** Scalp bandage is used for retaining addressing on the scalp.
   Method:
   - Apply the dressing and keep it in place with a ring pad.
   - Stand in front of the patient and apply the triangular bandage to the head, so that the point hangs down at the back of the neck, and the base comes on to the forehead. Fold in the base if necessary.
   - Carry the ends around the head to cross below the back of the head and take back to the front to tie off at the front. Fold the point up on the head and pin.
6. ***Other uses***
   - **Elbow bandage (Figs. 4.3.13A and B):** It comes under St John sling triangular bandage.

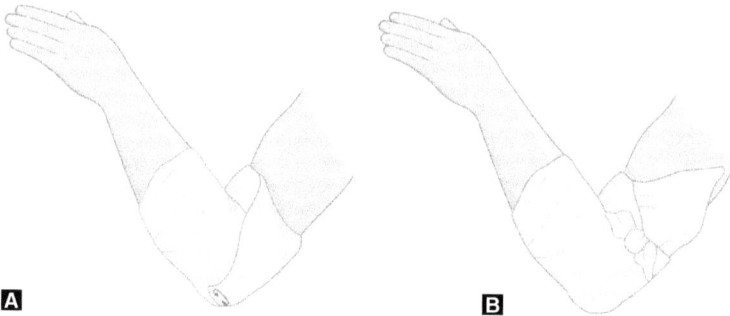

Figs. 4.3.13A and B: Application of sling bandage—elbow.

- **Shoulder bandage:** The bandage is retained in position by the sling, which may be either an open- or broad-fold triangular bandage.
- **Hip bandage (Figs. 4.3.14A to C):** A narrow fold triangular bandage is used to retain the hip bandage in place.
- **Bandage for back of chest:** Back of chest bandage is used for retaining dressing, which cover an extensive part of the chest, e.g., in case of burns. It consists of a triangular bandage and a narrow-fold bandage.
- **Bandage for chest:** Chest bandage is used for the same purpose as for 'back of chest'. Shifting the patient after bandaging is shown in **Figures 4.3.15A to D**.

Special Bandage: Tailed Bandages

Tailed bandages are used when roller bandages are not applicable. The tailed bandage includes:

- **T-bandage (Fig. 4.3.16A):** It is shaped like a "T" (and is made up of a vertical strip of material sewn or pinned to the center of a horizontal strip. This can be used to bandage the scalp, ear, eye, or perineum.
- **Double T-bandage (Fig. 4.3.16B):** To do this, sew two vertical strips of fabric, spaced about 4 inches apart, to the center of a horizontal strip. It can hold dressings for the perineum, back, or chest.
- **Four-tailed bandage (Fig. 4.3.16C):** It is a piece of material 4–6 inches wide and about 30 inches long, with each end cut about 12 or 14 inches down the middle, leaving the center piece about

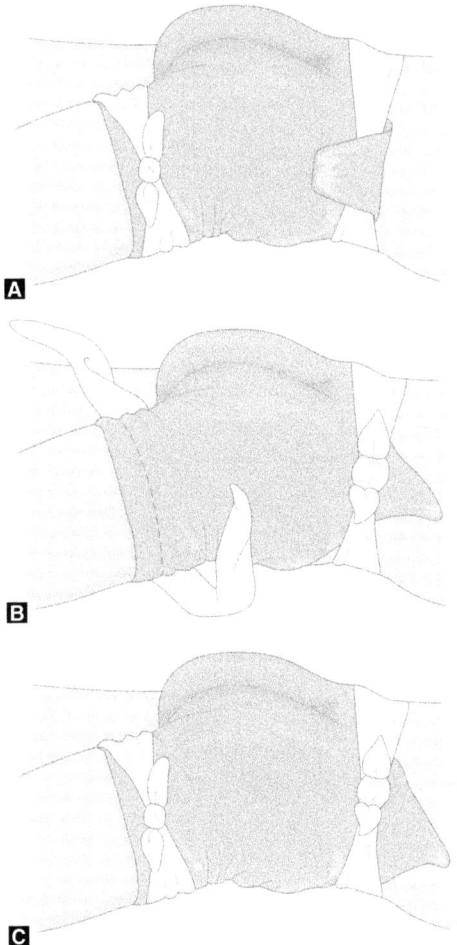

Figs. 4.3.14A to C: Bandaging fractured hip with triangular bandage.

12 or 14 inches long. This can be used to hold dressings on the jaw, nose, forehead, and back of the head.

- **Many-tailed bandage (Fig. 4.3.16D):** The only difference between a many-tailed bandage and a four-tailed bandage is that the ends are cut into the desired number of tails, which are approximately 16 inches in length and 20 inches for the uncut part.

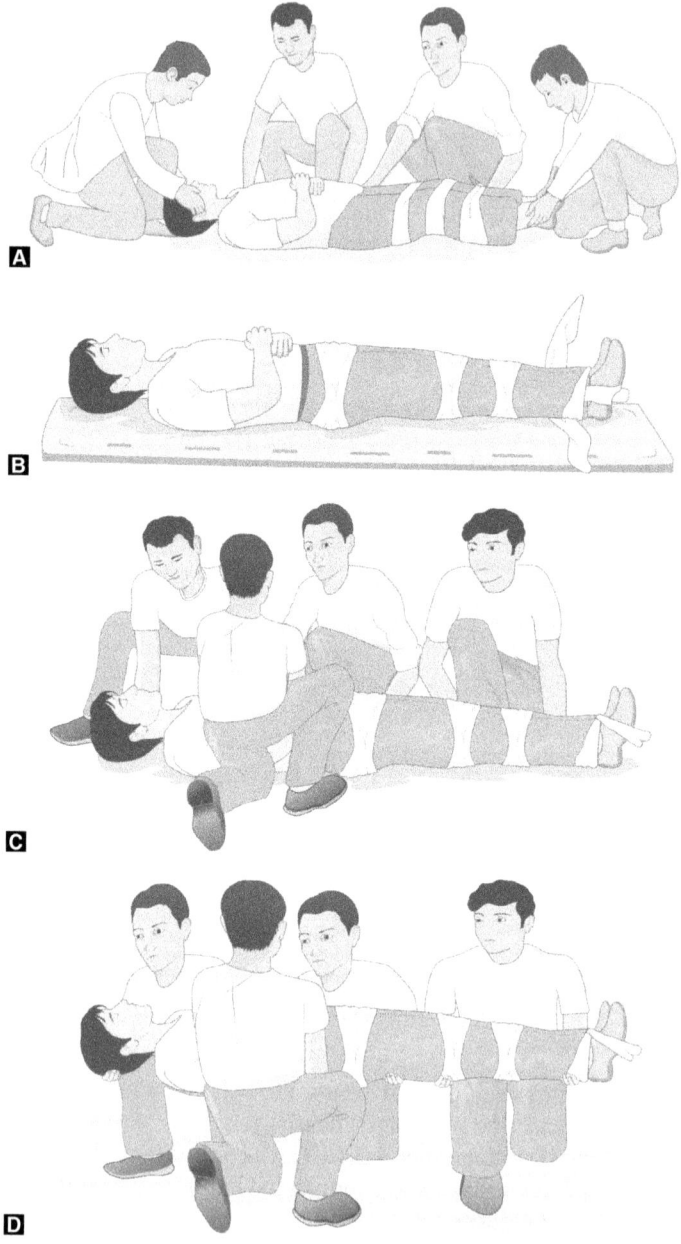

Figs. 4.3.15A to D: Shifting the patient after bandaging.

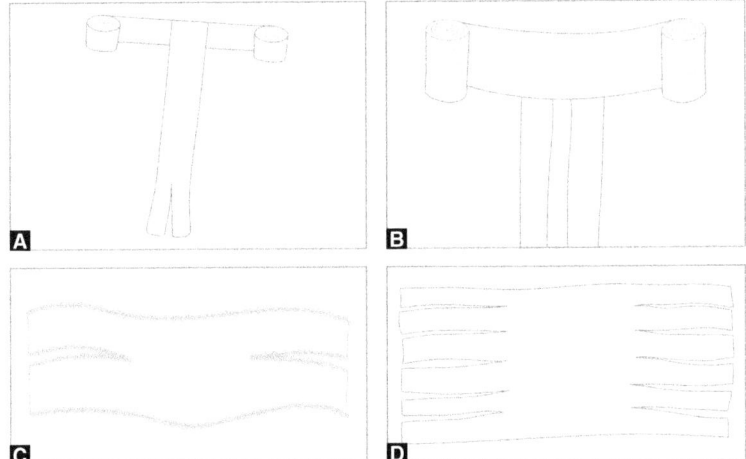

Figs. 4.3.16A to D: (A) T-bandage; (B) Double T-bandage; (C) Four-tailed bandage; (D) Many-tailed bandage.

Slings

Slings are used to support or to limit movement of the upper limb, in cases of injury or inflammation.

Types

Large Arm Sling

Large arm sling supports mainly the forearm and hand **(Fig. 4.3.17)**. It is sometimes used with splinting of the forearm. When applied, only the fingertips should show. The whole arm being well-supported, position of the hand should be slightly higher than the elbow. The knot should be in the hollow just above the clavicle on the injured side. The point is brought forward and secured with a safety pin to the front of the bandage. Check the color of the finger nails and if they are bluish, there is interference with the circulation and the bandage must be reapplied.

Collar and Cuff Sling

Collar and cuff sling is used to support the wrist in many cases of upper arm injury as shown in **Figure 4.3.18**. With the patient's forearm flexed and the finger's touching the opposite shoulder, a clove hitch made from a narrow bandage is placed round the wrist. The ends of the bandage pass round the neck and are tied in the hollow just above

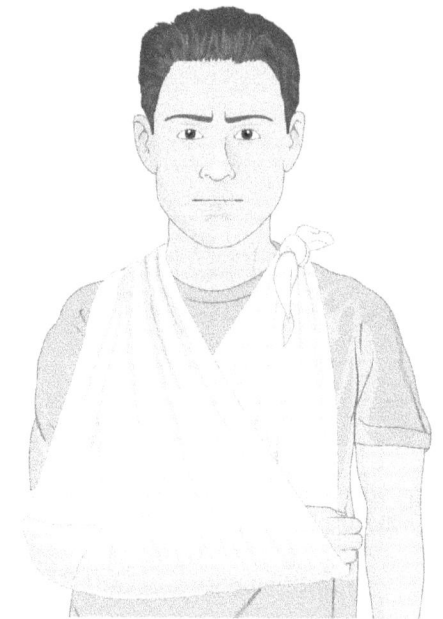

Fig. 4.3.17: Large arm sling.

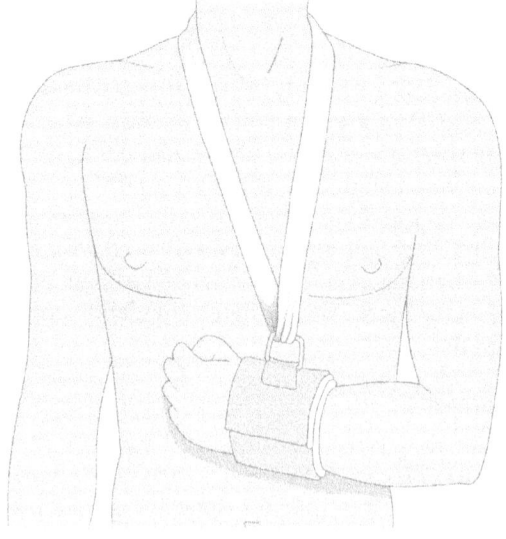

Fig. 4.3.18: Collar and cuff sling.

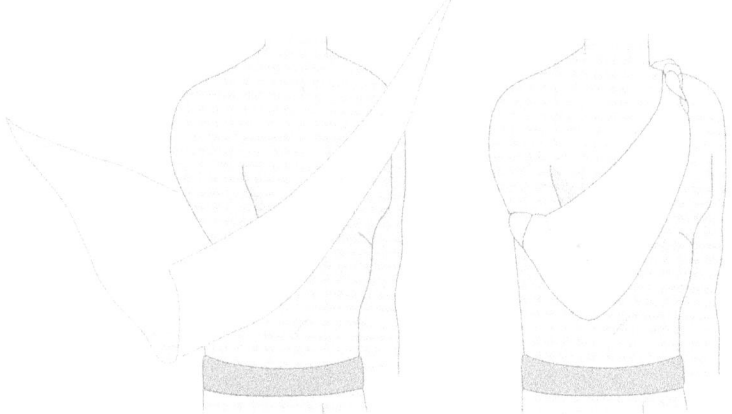

Fig. 4.3.19: St John sling.

the clavicle. To make a clove hitch, take a narrow bandage, make a loop; make a second loop and lay it on top of the first, then place the top loop behind the first without turning either loop.

St John Sling

St John sling supports the arm with the hand well raised and may be used for a fractured clavicle, or in shoulder injuries **(Fig. 4.3.19)**. The base of the bandage should be tucked well under the hand and one end brought round the back and the bandage tied just in front of the shoulder on the uninjured side. The point is folded over the forearm and the folded edge pinned to the bandage at the back.

Improvised Slings

When long sleeves are worn, the arm may be supported by pinning the sleeve to the clothing; or the lower edge of the coat may be turned up and pinned; or the arm may be supported inside a buttoned up coat, scarves, ties, belts, etc., may be improvised as slings as shown in **Figures 4.3.20A and B**.

Splints

A splint is a rigid appliance, usually made of wood or metal, which is tied to a fractured limb to support it and prevent movement from taking place at the site of fracture. Some first aid kits are supplied with wooden splints or metal splints made of aluminum or stout wire as

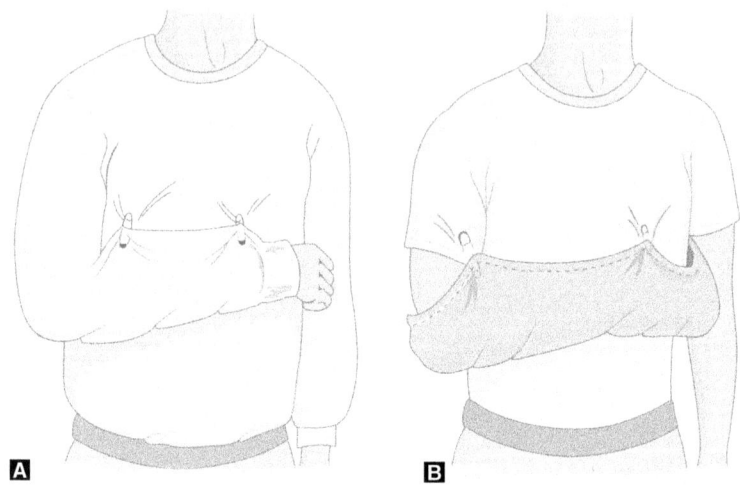

Figs. 4.3.20A and B: Improvised.

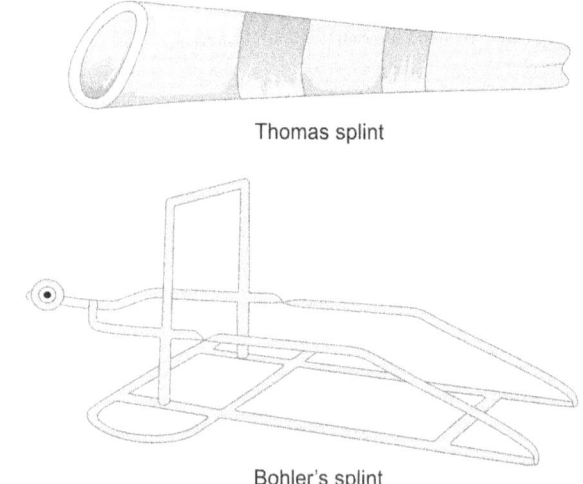

Thomas splint

Bohler's splint

Fig. 4.3.21: Types of splint.

shown in **Figure 4.3.21**. The latter could be cut to the required size and molded to the required shape.

However, splints can be improvised by using any article, which is rigid enough and of sufficient length for the purpose for which it is required. Rolled newspapers, magazines, etc., have been used for splinting in case of emergency. The body itself can be used for splinting purposes, e.g., a fractured arm can be strapped to the side of the chest to immobilize it, a fractured leg can be tied to the other leg, etc.

Using a Splint

If a splint is not used properly, it may cause damage. Therefore, remember the following points when using a splint:

- Make sure that the splint is well padded. This is particularly important when splints are improvised from pieces of wood, which are uneven.
- Make sure that the splint is sufficiently long to immobilize the joints above and below the fracture.
- Make sure that the bandage is used to secure the parts. The splint should have the knot tied on the splint and not on the fleas.

REVIEW QUESTIONS

LONG ESSAYS

1. Define bandages and explain the purpose and principles in details.
2. Describe the various bandaging patterns.
3. Define slings and explain the types of slings.

SHORT ESSAYS

1. Explain the uses of triangular bandages.
2. Describe the steps for application of capeline bandage.
3. Splint.
4. Tailed bandages.
5. Roller bandages.

Transportation of Injured Persons

CHAPTER 5

CHAPTER OUTLINE

- Methods of Transportation
  - Single Rescuer: Cradle Method, Human Crutch, Pick-a-Back, Reverse Pick-a-Back, Fireman's Lift and Carry
  - Two or More Rescuer: Hand Seats, Fore and AFT Carry Method, Chair Method, Wheelchair Method, Stretchers

INTRODUCTION

Transporting severely injured people to the hospital is a critical step in first aid. Depending on the type of injuries, the patient should be transported in the best position for their injuries. The patient should be moved by appropriately trained support personnel who are equipped with the necessary equipment to stabilize vital structures and prevent further harm.

TRANSPORT OF INJURED PERSONS (TO BE DEMONSTRATED)

An injured person can be moved to shelter by any of the following methods:
- Support by a single helper.
- Hand seats.
- Stretcher.
- Wheeled transport.

METHODS OF TRANSPORTATION

The method(s) adopted will depend upon the following factors:
- Nature of the injury.
- Severity of the injury.
- Number of helpers available.

CHAPTER 5: Transportation of Injured Persons

- Distance to shelter.
- Nature of the route to be traversed.

Method of Transportation for Single First Aider

Cradle Method (Fig. 5.1A)
- To be used only in the case of light casualties or children.
- Lift the casualty by passing one of the arms well beneath casualty's two knees, and the other around back.

Human Crutch (Fig. 5.1B)
Standing at the injured side, except where there is injury to an upper limb, assist the casualty by putting arm round his/her waist, grasping the clothing at hip and placing the arm round neck, holding his/her hand with bearer's free hand. If casualty's upper limb is injured and other hand is free, the casualty may gain additional help from a staff or walking stick.

Pick-a-Back (Fig. 5.1C)
If the casualty is conscious and able to hold on, he/she may be carried in the ordinary 'pick-a-back' fashion. The injured person is lifted by

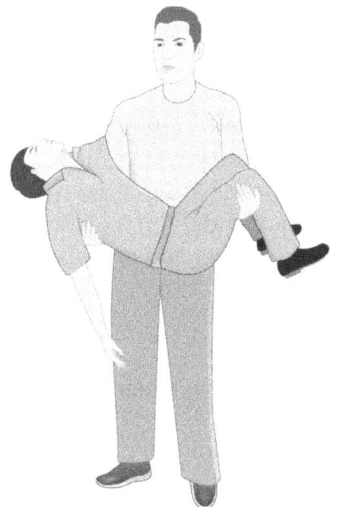

Fig. 5.1A: Cradle method.

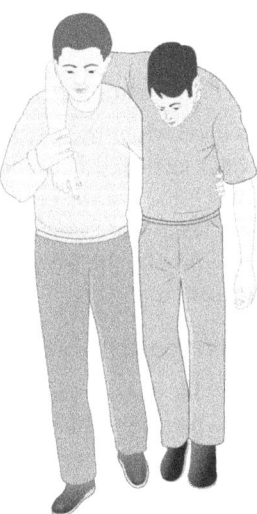

Fig. 5.1B: Human crutch.

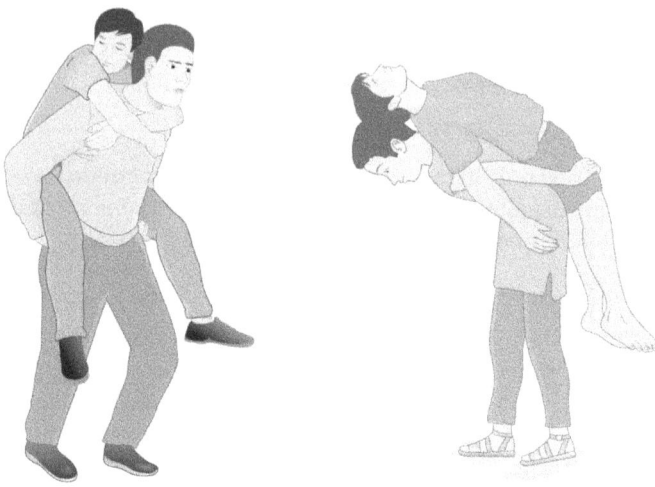

Fig. 5.1C: Pick-a-back.   **Fig. 5.1D:** Reverse pick-a-back.

the rescuer onto his or her back. The victim grips the rescuer's waist and neck with his legs and arms. The rescuer supports the injured person by passing both hands behind and back or under the knees.

Reverse Pick-a-Back (Fig. 5.1D)

This is used when the casualty is too heavy to be lifted. The patient leans back against the rescuer back in backward position, the rescuer supports him. The rescuer wraps both hands around the injured person's waist and passes both hands backwards. The rescuer leans forward and lifts the injured person off their feet and onto the back of the rescuer.

Fireman's Lift and Carry (Fig. 5.1E)

Fireman's lift and carry method should be used only when the casualty is not too heavy for the bearer.
- Assist the victim in rising to an upright position.
- Grasp his/her right wrist with left hand.
- Bend down with head under his/her extended right arm, so that right shoulder is level with the lower part of casualty's abdomen and place the right arm between or round his/her legs.

CHAPTER 5: Transportation of Injured Persons | 117

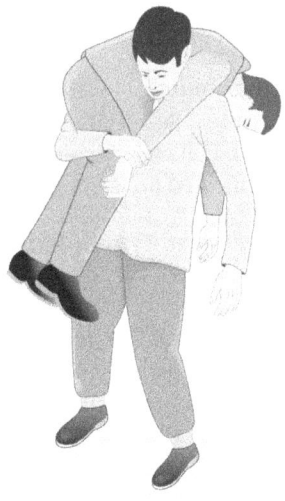

Fig. 5.1E: Fireman's lift and carry.

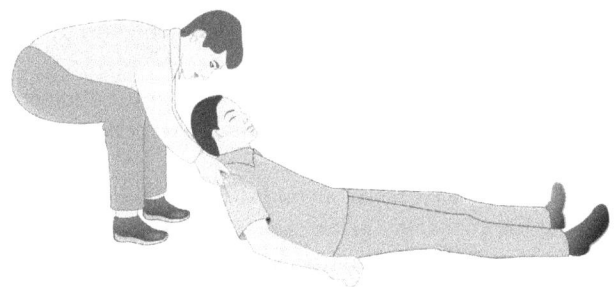

Fig. 5.1F: Drag method.

- While taking the weight on right shoulder, rise to the erect position.
- Pull the casualty across both shoulders and transfer his/her right wrist to right hand, so leaving left hand free.

Drag Method (Fig. 5.1F)

Drag method involves pulling the casualty along the ground without lifting. It should only be used where a casualty is unable to stand and must be moved quickly from a source of danger in the following ways:

- Fold the casualty's arms across his/her chest and crouch behind head; place hands under his/her shoulders, grasp the armpits and cradle the head on forearms.
- Pull him/her along the ground.
- If the casualty is wearing a jacket or coat, unbutton it and pull it back up under the head. Pull him/her along the ground in the same way with the head supported on the coat.

Method of Transportation for Two or More Rescuer

Hand Seats

- **Four-handed seat (Fig. 5.2A):** This seat is used when the casualty can assist the bearer by using one or both arms:
  - Two bearers face each other behind the casualty and grasp their left wrists with their right hands and each other's right wrists with their left hands and stoop down.
  - The casualty is instructed to place one arm round the neck of each bearer, so that he/she may raise himself/herself to sit on their hands and be steady during transport.
  - The bearers rise together and stop off, the bearer on the right hand side of the casualty with the right foot, and the left hand bearer with the left foot.
- **Two-handed seat (Fig. 5.2B):** This seat is mostly used to carry a casualty who is unable to assist the bearers by using his/her arms:
  - Two bearers face each other and stoop (not kneel) one on each side of the casualty. Each bearer passes their forearm nearest to the casualty's head and back just below the shoulders, and, if possible, takes hold of clothing.
  - Both rescuer slightly raise the casualty's back and then pass their other forearms under the middle of his/her thigh and clasp their hands; the bearer on the left of the casualty with the palm upwards and holding a folded handkerchief to prevent hurting by the finger nails; bearer on right of the casualty with palm downwards.
  - The bearers rise together and step off, the right-hand bearer with the right foot and the left hand bearer with the left foot.
  - In all cases of carrying by hand seats, the bearers walk with the crossover step and not by side paces.

CHAPTER 5: Transportation of Injured Persons

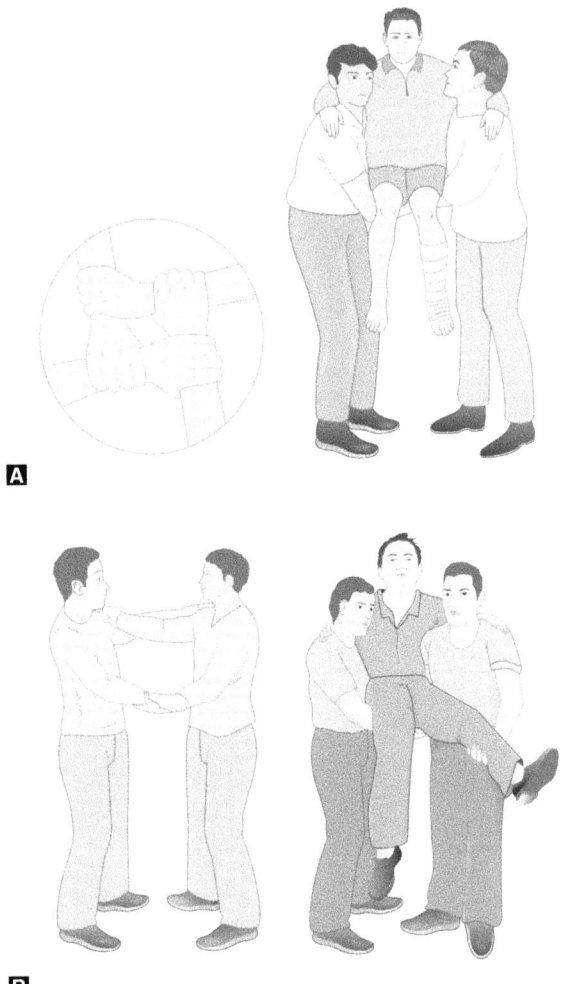

Figs. 5.2A and B: (A) Four handed seat; (B) Two handed seat.

Fore-and-Aft Carry Method (Fig. 5.3A)

Fore-and-aft carry method can be used to place the casualty on a chair or a carrying chair. This method should not be used if the upper limb is injured. The method is as follows:
- Supporting the casualty on both sides, both first aiders should help the casualty to sit up and fold his/her arms across chest.

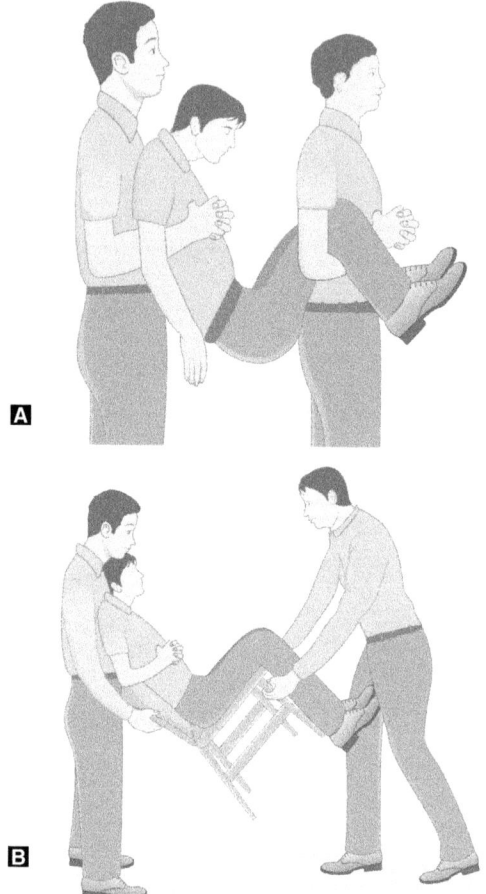

Figs. 5.3A and B: (A) Fore-and-aft method; (B) Chair method.

- One rescuer stoops at the back of the casualty and grasps the casualty's wrists by reaching under the casualty's arms.
- The second rescuer stand between the casualty's legs grasping them underneath the knees.
- Both rescuers work together to lift the casualty onto the chair or stretcher.

Chair Method (Fig. 5.3B)

When a conscious casualty with no serious injuries is to be moved up or downstairs or along passageways the casualty can be seated on

an ordinary chair and carried by two people. However, the passages must be cleared of any obstructions or dangers such as loose matting before one start. The method is as follows:
- Test the chair to ensure that it is strong enough to support the casualty, then sit him/her down and secure in position with broad bandages. Stand facing each other, one in front of the chair and one in behind.
- The person behind the chair should support the back of the chair and the casualty; the other person should hold the chair by the front legs. Slowly tilt the chair backwards to seat the casualty securely, then lift together.
- With the casualty facing forwards, move slowly along the passage or stairs.
- If space permits, the bearer can both stand facing the side of the chair each supporting the back and the top of a front leg.

Wheelchair Method

Wheelchair bound casualties can be transported by adapting the chair method where they sit in the following way:
- Locate the brakes and apply securely.
- Make the casualty to sit well back in the chair.
- Examine the wheelchair to find out which parts are fixed—arm rests and side supports are often removable and will detach if the bearer use them to lift the chair. Supporting the chair from either side, lift by holding the fixed parts, never by the wheels.
- Carry the chair as described in chair method.

Stretchers

Stretchers are used to carry a seriously ill or injured casualty to an ambulance or similar shelter to minimize the risk of further injury. The stretchers in general use include the following:
- Standard stretcher
- Scoop stretcher
- Trolley bed
- Utila folding stretcher
- Carrying sheet
- Carrying chair
- Neil-Robertson stretcher
- Paraguard stretcher

Most stretchers can be used to transport casualties with any injury and should be rigid enough to carry casualties with a suspected spine fracture without additional boards. All equipment must be tested before it is used.

Testing a Stretcher

To ensure that a stretcher is capable of taking the weight of a casualty, one person should lie on the stretcher and each end of the stretcher should be lifted in turn. Then both ends should be lifted at the same time.

> **Note:**
> If possible, test the stretcher before leaving an ambulance station and not in front of a casualty.

Opening the Stretcher

- Place the stretcher on its side with its runners towards the bearer and the studs or buckles securing straps upper most. Unfasten any straps.
- Push the traverses fully open with foot. Whilst placing the stretcher upright on either end.

Closing the Stretcher

- Turn the stretcher on its side so that the runners are facing the bearer and the studs or buckles that fasten the straps at the top are facing the bearer. Push the joints of the traverses inwards with heel to release them.
- Push the poles together, pulling the canvas out from between them. Fold the canvas neatly on to the poles and secure with the straps.

Different Types of Stretchers

Standard Stretcher (Fig. 5.4A)

- The 'standard' or Furley stretcher consists of poles, handles, traverses, runners and a canvas bed.
- The traverses are joined so that the stretcher can be opened and closed.
- When closed, the poles lie close together with the canvas bed folded on top. This is then kept in position by two transverse straps.
- If slings are carried, they are laid along the canvas held by the straps.

Scoop Stretcher (Fig. 5.4B)

The scoop or orthopedic stretcher is an adjustable stretcher used to lift casualties on to an ambulance trolley bed without altering the position in which they were found. It is used to carry a casualty any distance. The length can be adjusted to suit any size of casualty and because he/she does not have to be moved, it is particularly useful for picking up a casualty with a suspected spinal fracture or internal injuries. Hard objects from the casualty's pocket must be removed while shifting. The method is as follows:

- Bring the stretcher to the casualty's side and adjust the length.
- Uncouple both ends of the stretcher and gently slip each half of the stretcher under the casualty; rejoin the head sections.
- Place the head pad in position.
- While one first aider stays at the head, the other should rejoin the foot section. Secure the head pad to the stretcher.
- Working from either side of the stretcher, lift it and place the casualty on the trolley bed. Uncouple the stretcher and remove it.

Trolley Bed (Fig. 5.4C)

Trolley bed is a fully adjustable stretcher bed on wheels. It is made of light metal and is carried in many ambulances. Trolley beds should always be kept prepared for immediate use. A canvas sheet from a pole and canvas stretcher is laid on the stretcher bed and two blankets are placed on top.

Utila Folding Stretcher (Fig. 5.4D)

Utila folding stretcher is a lightweight version of the standard stretcher. It has light metal poles with telescopic handles and a canvas or plastic bed. The folding stretcher is available in two versions. One folds in the same way as the standard stretcher; the other folds in half at the center and so takes up less space.

Carrying Sheet (Fig. 5.4E)

Carrying sheet is used during emergency evacuation during hazardous situations. The carrying sheet has ten large wrap around hand loops, it can be folded and enclosed in carry bad.

Carrying Chair (Fig. 5.4F)

A carrying chair is used to transport a sick or injured person away from an accident or hazardous location. The victim is seated in a chair and is being carried by two rescuers. This is the most practical method for transporting a casualty upstairs.

Neil Robertson Stretcher (Fig. 5.4G)

The Neil Robertson stretcher is intended to transport an injured person from places where doors, hatches, or other access points are too small to accommodate standard stretchers. Mainly used on a ship, examples of these small spaces include the boiler room, cargo holds, pump rooms, and engine rooms. When not in use or when fitting into tight spaces, the Neil Robertson stretcher can be easily folded as it is flexible yet semi-rigid canvas construction. The stretcher straps are designed so that when they are wrapped around the victim, they enclose them like a mummy and provide enough support.

Paraguard Stretcher (Fig. 5.4H)

The Paraguard stretcher is used to move injured people from high buildings, underground spaces, high altitude areas, and confined spaces. Examples include lifting casualty by helicopter from snow area or mountain terrain. This stretcher can be used by a single rescuer and is very helpful in keeping the patient immobile while moving. While being transported, the casualty can be lifted either vertically or horizontally.

Transporting Casualty to Stretcher

An important step in emergency management is lifting the casualty onto a stretcher. Maximum caution must be used when lifting in order to prevent the casualty's condition from worsening. The following steps may be taken depending on the availability of responders or manpower **(Figs. 5.5A to D)**:

- ❖ Each responder must knelt on the knee closest to the victim's feet.
- ❖ The rescuers must lift the patient on command of the person at the head.
- ❖ Once the rescuers receive the command, they should lift the casualty up and rest him/her on their knees.
- ❖ The rescuers must place the casualty down on stretcher after command by the person at the head.
- ❖ Rescuers must always keep in mind that unnecessary movement of the casualty increases the risk of further harm or complications.

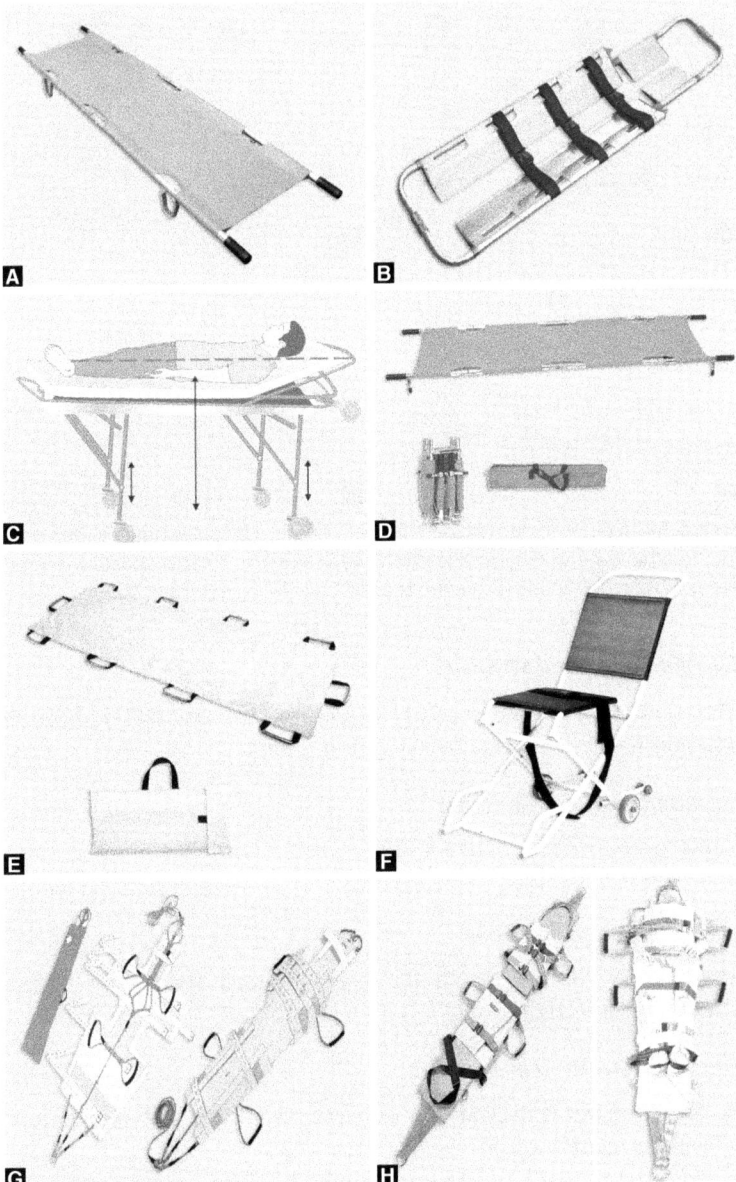

Figs. 5.4A to H: Types of stretchers: (A) Standard stretcher; (B) Scoop stretcher; (C) Trolley bed; (D) Utila folding stretcher; (E) Carrying sheet; (F) Carrying chair; (G) Neil Robertson stretcher; (H) Paraguard stretcher.

SECTION 2: First Aid Management

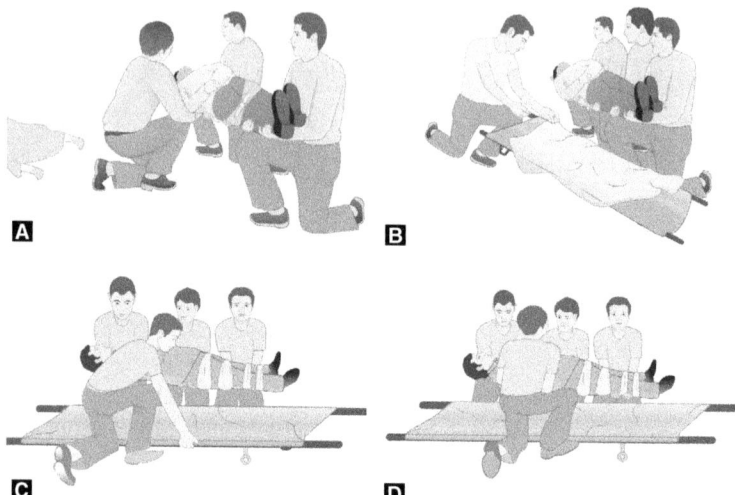

Figs. 5.5A to D: Lifting an accident victim: (A) Lifted by three bearers (helpers); (B) Stretcher is holded by one helper to place a victim; (C) Stretcher is arranged below to place a victim; (D) Victim is to be placed on stretcher by four bearers.

Carrying a Loaded Stretcher

The number of people needed to carry the stretcher will determine whether it will be carried by two or four people.

Lowering a Loaded Stretcher

The bearers will stoop gently and lower the stretcher to the ground and then rise together.

Lifting a Loaded Stretcher

The bearers will pick the stretcher steadily together by keeping the stretcher at a straight level.

Loading a Stretcher in Ambulance

- ❖ The stretcher is moved one step away from the ambulance door with its head lowered.
- ❖ The stretcher will be raised evenly to the level of the berth to be loaded, and the casualty will be loaded head first while loading **(Fig. 5.6)**.

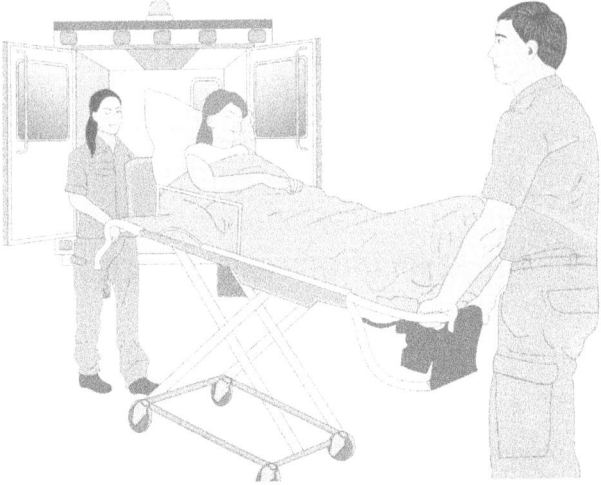

Fig. 5.6: Loading head first in an ambulance.

- The front bearers place the runners in the grooves and then assist the rear bearers to slide the stretcher into its place and secure it.
- If slings are used, they should be kept with their stretcher.

REVIEW QUESTIONS

LONG ESSAYS

1. List the various methods of transportation of injured person's and explain Fireman's lift and carry method.
2. Explain the different stretcher methods of transportation.
3. Describe methods of transporting a casualty by single first aider.

SHORT ESSAYS

1. Steps for loading a casualty in ambulance.
2. Difference between pick-a-back and reverse pick-a-back method.
3. Explain hand seats methods.
4. Scoop stretcher method.
5. Fore-and-aft carry method.

Respiratory Emergencies and Basic CPR

CHAPTER 6

6.1: RESPIRATORY EMERGENCIES

Chapter Outline

- Asphyxia
- Choking
- External Obstruction
- Suffocation
- Asthma
- Smoke Inhalation
- Drowning
- Hanging, Strangling and Throttling

INTRODUCTION

Respiratory emergencies includes all emergencies health problem associated with airways, thoracic and pulmonary system. This chapter discuss about respiratory emergencies such as Asphyxia, Choking, External obstruction, Suffocation, Asthma, smoke inhalation, drowning, hanging, strangling and throttling (refer **Table 6.1.1** for first aid measures in special cases).

ASPHYXIA

Asphyxia is a potentially fatal condition, which occurs if enough oxygen is not available to the tissues of the body. Such deficiency may be due to an insufficient amount of oxygen in the air breathed in or any interference with, or injury to the respiratory system. Without an adequate supply of oxygen, the tissues deteriorate very rapidly. Vital nerve cells in the brain can die after only 3 minutes without oxygen.

Definition

Asphyxia is a condition that occurs due to lack of oxygen supply in respired air or any interference with the respiratory system, leading to oxygen deprivation in the organs and tissue causing unconsciousness or death.

CHAPTER 6: Respiratory Emergencies and Basic CPR

Table 6.1.1: First aid in special cases.

Respiratory emergencies	First aid measures
Drowning	• Perform artificial respiration • Instruct bystanders to remove clothing of the victim as far as practicable • Wrap the casualty in dry blanket or dry clothing
Strangulation	Cut and remove the band/rope constricting the throat
Hanging	• Grasp the lower limbs and raise the body • Free the neck by loosening or cutting the rope • Do not wait for policemen • Keep all materials as it is, later for evidence
Choking	• To dislodge the obstruction, bend the casualty's head and shoulder forward • In the case of a small child hold him/her upside down and thump his/her back hard between the shoulder blades • If this is not necessary, encourage vomiting by passing two fingers right to the back of the casualty's throat
Swelling of tissues within the throat	• If breathing has not ceased or when it has been restored give ice to suck, if failing, ice cold water to sip • Butter, olive oil or medicinal paraffin may also be given
Suffocation by smoke	• Tie a towel, handkerchief or cloth, preferable wet, over your mouth and nose • Maintain a lower posture and remove the casualty as quickly as possible
Suffocation by poisonous gas	• Before entering the suspected space, take a deep breath and hold it • Ensure a free circulation of air by opening or if necessary, by braking doors or windows • If the gas is lighter than air maintain lower posture • If heavier, remain in the upright position • Remove the casualty as quickly as possible • In cases of no ventilation and deadly gas, a suitable gas mask must be worn • An additional safety precaution is a lifeline

Causes of Asphyxia

- Conditions affecting the casualty's airway and lungs:
  - *Obstructed airway:* Due to the tongue falling into the back of the throat in an unconscious casualty; food, vomit or other foreign matter present in the airway, or swelling of the tissues in the throat resulting from scalds, stings or infection.
  - Fluid in the air passages.
  - Compression of the windpipe by handing or strangulation.
  - Compression of the chest caused by a fall of earth or sand being crushed against a wall or barrier, or pressure from a crowd.
  - Injury to the lungs.
  - Injury to the chest wall, e.g., a stove-in chest.
  - Fits preventing adequate breathing.
- Conditions affecting the brain or nerves, which control respiration include:
  - Electrical injury.
  - Poisoning.
  - Paralysis caused by a stroke or injury to the spinal cord.
- Conditions affecting the amount of oxygen in the blood include:
  - Air containing insufficient oxygen: Gas or smoke-filled buildings or shafts and tunnels.
  - Change in atmospheric pressure: High altitudes, in depressurized aircraft or after deep-sea diving.
- Conditions preventing the use of oxygen in the body include:
  - Carbon monoxide poisoning.
  - Cyanide poisoning

Signs and Symptoms

Early stage	*Later stage*
• Dizziness and weakness. • Shortness of breath. • Rapid pulse. • Partial loss of consciousness. • Swelling of the veins of the neck. • Congestion of the face with blueness of cheeks and lips.	• The lips, nose, ears, fingers and toes are bluish gray. • Breathing intermittent or absent. • Pulse slow and irregular. • Complete loss of consciousness.

GENERAL RULES FOR MANAGEMENT OF ASPHYXIA

- Remove the cause, if possible or the casualty from the cause.
- Ensure that there is a free passage for air. In an unconscious person the tongue may fall back and obstruct the air passages. This possibility should be kept constantly in mind if the casualty is lying on his/her back.
- Apply artificial respiration immediately. Even in seconds' count. Artificial respiration must be continued until natural breathing is restored, if necessary for a long time unless a doctor decides that further efforts will be of no avail.
- Place the patient in recovery position, when pulse and breathing return.
- Check the breathing pattern, pulse rate and level of unconsciousness every 10 minutes interval.
- Utilize any help available to:
  - Provide warmth, e.g., blankets.
  - Provide shelter from the elements.

CHOKING

Definition

Choking occurs when the airway is partially or totally obstructed by something, which in the act of swallowing, goes into windpipe rather than down the food passage. Choking require immediate attention as it can cause blocking of airflow leading to death.

Causes

- Chewing food inadequately.
- Swallowing food in hurry.
- Speaking while eating.
- Putting objects inside the mouth (In children).

Signs and Symptoms

Partial airway obstruction	Total airway obstruction
• Labored, gasping or noisy breathing. • Coughing. • Making "crowning" noise. • Escape of some air from mouth. • Anxiety or agitation.	• Unable to produce effective cough, breathe or speak. • Constant efforts to breathe from within by drawing spaces between the ribs and above the collarbones. • The casualty can be seen clutching the throat with both hands.

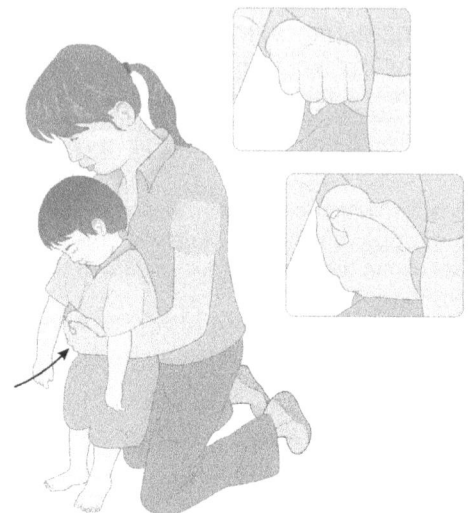

Fig. 6.1.1: Heimlich Maneuver on child.

Management of Choking

Heimlich Maneuver/Abdominal Thrusts

- ❖ Stand behind the patient and place foot slightly in front of the other. In case of child, kneel down behind the child **(Figure 6.1.1)**.
- ❖ Wrap both arms around the waist and tip the patient forward slightly.
- ❖ Make a fist with one hand and position it slightly above the person's navel.
- ❖ Grasp the fist with the other hand and press hard into the abdomen with a quick upward thrust.
- ❖ Perform between six and 10 abdominal thrusts until the blockage is dislodged.

First Aid Measures for Partial and total Airway Obstruction

Partial airway obstruction	Total airway obstruction
• Ask the patient "are you choking"? (If patient is able to answer, it is a partial airway obstruction).	Back blow method • Give 5 back blows **(Figure 6.1.2A)** between the patient's shoulder blades. • Check in between each blow to see if item has been dislodged.

CHAPTER 6: Respiratory Emergencies and Basic CPR

- Stay with the patient.
- Encourage to cough and expel the foreign body.
- If unable to expel out the foreign body, call ambulance.
- Do not give back blow.

- In case of baby, place the baby face down on your lap for the back blows **(Figure 6.1.2B)**.

If back blows is unsuccessful, follow chest trusts method:

- Wrap both arms around the patient, at chest level **(Figure 6.1.2A)**
- Place one fist with the thumb on side against middle of the breastbone.
- Grasp that fist with your other hand and give up to five separate inward and upward thrusts.
- Check between each chest trust to see if the item has been dislodged.
- Place a baby face upwards on a firm surface and give up to five sharp chest thrusts just below the nipple line, checking between each thrust.
- If patient is unconscious, perform CPR.
- Call an ambulance.

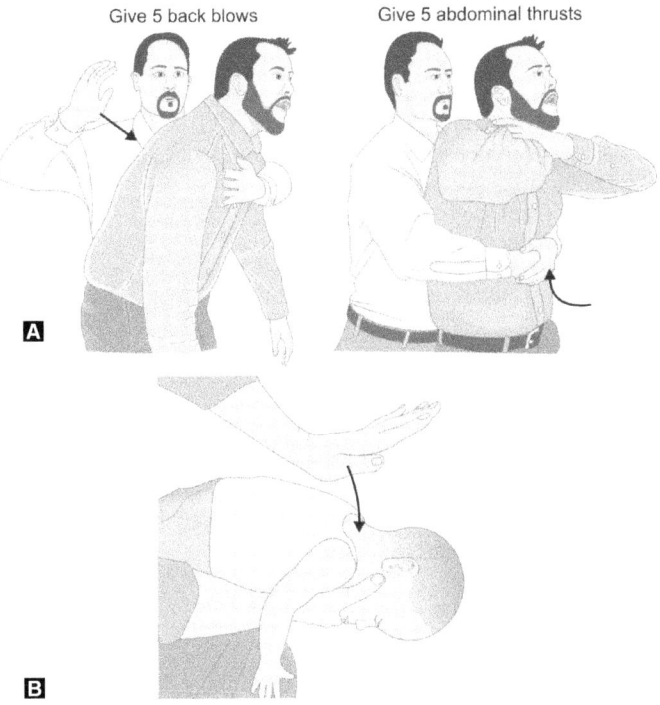

Figs. 6.1.2A and B: (A) Five and five approach; (B) Back blow method on infant.

EXTERNAL OBSTRUCTION

Definition

External obstruction results when air is prevented from reaching the air passages by an external obstruction such as a plastic bag, soft pillow or a fall of sand. A baby may be suffocated by lying face down on a pillow or cushion.

Signs and Symptoms

- Difficulty in breathing—the rate and depth of breathing increases.
- Breathing may become noisy with snoring or gurgling.

MANAGEMENT OF EXTERNAL OBSTRUCTION
- Immediately remove any obstruction and move the casualty in a open space area.
- If casualty is conscious and breathing, reassure and observe.
- If casualty is unconscious, open airway and check breathing. Perform CPR if required and place his/her in the recovery position.
- Seek medical aid, if in doubt about his/her condition, arrange transportation to hospital:
  - Possible frothing at the mouth.
  - Bluish coloration of face, lips and fingernails (cyanosis).
  - Confusion.
  - Lowering of level of responsiveness.
  - Possible unconsciousness.
  - Breathing may stop.

SUFFOCATION

Definition

Suffocation is the act of blocking airflow entering the lungs by closing a person's nose and mouth simultaneously. This can be caused by irritant gases, smokes or fumes, pillow or plastic bag pressed on the face. Suffocation can lead to death.

Suffocation by Smoke

Signs and Symptoms
- Vision difficulty
- Chest tightness

- Coughing, wheezing and hoarseness
- Difficulty in breathing
- Headache
- Fainting
- Abdominal pain

MANAGEMENT OF SUFFOCATION BY SMOKE
- Find and remove the patient from smoke as soon as possible.
- Tie a towel, handkerchief or cloth, preferably wet, over your mouth and nose.
- Let the patient sit in upright position.
- Loosen clothing around the neck.
- If casualty stop breathing, perform CPR.

Suffocation by Poisonous Gas

Common Poisonous Gas that Causes Suffocation

- **Gases lighter than air:** Carbon monoxide (found as a result of combustion in car exhaust vapors and in household coal gas and as a result of incomplete combustion, i.e., charcoal stoves and as white damp in coal mines), ammonia and methane or marsh gas (found as its name implies in marshes and as fire damp in coal mines).
- **Gases heavier than air:** Carbon dioxide (found in the black damp of coal mines), sulfuretted hydrogen (found in sewer gas), carbon tetrachloride (vapor from fire extinguishers), methyl bromide (vapor from leaking refrigerators and varieties of compressed gas used for cooking and lighting).

MANAGEMENT OF SUFFOCATION BY POISONOUS GAS
- Before entering any closed space known or suspected to contain poisonous gas of any kind, take a deep breath and hold it.
- Ensure a free circulation of air by opening or if necessary, by breaking doors or windows.
- If the gas is lighter than air, keep low, if heavier, remain in the upright position.
- Remove the casualty as quickly as possible.
- In cases where ventilation is not possible, and the character of the gas is known to be deadly a suitable gas mask be worn.

SECTION 2: First Aid Management

ASTHMA

Definition

Asthma is a medical condition affecting the airway **(Fig. 6.1.3)**. Asthma attack is caused by inflammation of the air passage, causing difficulty in breathing out. Narrowed airways are caused by muscle spasm, swelling and increased mucus production.

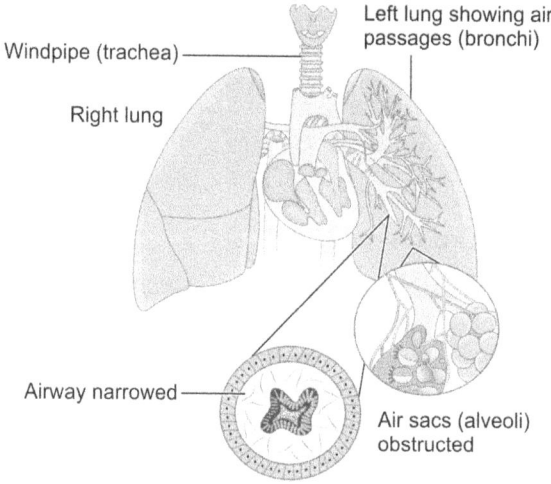

Fig. 6.1.3: Respiratory system showing narrowed airway and obstructed alveoli.

Causes of Asthma Attack

- Chest infection
- **Allergy:** Pollens, dust, drugs, fumes etc.
- Smoke
- Cold air or exercise.

Signs and Symptoms

- Difficulty in breathing.
- Difficulty in speaking more than a few words.
- Persistent cough (moist and rattling).
- Wheezing
- Sudden loss of consciousness and stoppage of breathing.
- Poor skin color, especially blueness of lips and fingertips.

CHAPTER 6: Respiratory Emergencies and Basic CPR 137

MANAGEMENT OF ASTHMA
- Help the patient to rest.
- Help the patient sit in a comfortable position by sitting upright, leaning forward with arms resting on a table.
- Call an ambulance.
- If spacer is available with the patient, give 6 puffs of the medication and then repeat this dose after about 6 minutes.
- Continue to assist the patient with 6 puffs every 6 minutes until an ambulance arrives.

SMOKE INHALATION

A fire uses up oxygen in the atmosphere so the oxygen level in a burning room is low and asphyxia may result. Smoke may irritate the throat, which can go into spasm and close the airway. In addition, the plastic coverings and foam padding of modern furnishings, when burning, often give off highly toxic fumes, which can be fatal.

Signs and Symptoms

- Same as signs and symptoms of asphyxia.
- Casualty may be scorched or burned (scorched hair in the nostrils is a valuable warning sign).
- Signs and symptoms of shock cause by burns.

MANAGEMENT
Aim: Restore fresh air and adequate breathing.
- Call the emergency services immediately.
- Remove the casualty from the fire and smoke if it is sure there are no toxic fumes present.
- Try to extinguish the fire.
- Arrange for transportation of patient to the hospital.

DROWNING

Drowning causes asphyxia by water entering to the lungs or by causing the throat to go into spasm thereby constricting the air passage.

Signs and Symptoms

- Similar to general signs and symptoms of asphyxia.
- Froth around the casualty's lips, mouth and nostrils.

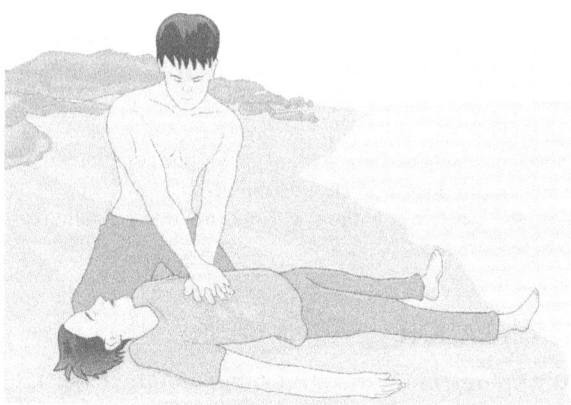

Fig. 6.1.4: CPR on drowning casualty.

- Hypothermia
- Injuries to head and neck
- Internal injuries—broken bones, soft tissue injuries, internal bleeding.
- Lungs congestion.

> **MANAGEMENT**
> - Follow DRCAB method.
> - Call emergency service/ambulance immediately.
> - If patient is unconscious and not breathing-perform CPR **(Fig. 6.1.4)**.
> - If patient in unconscious and breathing—place patient in recovery position.
> - Once patient gain consciousness, roll onto their side to ease breathing, clear airway and ensure they don't choke on any water regurgitation.
> - Cover casualty with warm clothes and blankets to prevent hypothermia (Change wet clothes if possible)

Prevention Measures for Drowning

- Fence the pool.
- Teach kids to swim.
- Children must be always under adult supervision while playing in the pool.
- Ensure individuals wear floatation device while swimming.
- Take safety precautions (no running, no diving) at all times.

HANGING, STRANGLING AND THROTTLING

Pressure on the outside of the neck by hanging, strangling or throttling squeezed the airway shut and blocks off the flow of air to the lungs:
- **Hanging:** It involves suspension of the body by the neck from nose.
- **Strangling:** It involves cutting off the air supply by a tight constriction around the neck.
- **Throttling:** It involves cutting off the air supply by intentional squeezing of the person's throat, as in an assault.

The first two conditions may occur accidentally, e.g., a tie may become caught in machinery.

Signs and Symptoms

- Body may still be suspended
- Similar with general signs and symptoms of asphyxia
- Congestion of the face and neck with the veins becoming prominent
- Constriction may still be visible around neck (e.g., scarf), or it may be hidden in the folds of the skin (e.g., wire)
- There may be marks around the casualty's throat or neck, where a constriction has been removed

MANAGEMENT

Aim: Restore adequate breathing and arrange transportation to hospital.
- Remove the constriction from around the casualty's neck immediately, supporting the weight of his/her body if he/she is hanging. If there is a knot, cut below it (a knot is difficult to cut, and it may be useful evidence).
- If the casualty is unconscious, open his/her airway and check breathing. Perform CPR, if required and place the casualty in the recovery position.
- Arrange the transportation to hospital.

Note: Seek medical aid even if recovery seems complete.

REVIEW QUESTIONS

LONG ESSAYS

1. Define asphyxia. Describe the first aid management for asphyxia.
2. What is choking? Explain first aid management for partial and total airway obstruction.

3. Define suffocation. Discuss first aid management for suffocation by poisonous gas.

SHORT ESSAYS

1. Describe about drowning and its management.
2. First aid management of carbon monoxide poisoning.
3. First aid management for Asthma attack.
4. Define hanging, strangling and throttling. Mention first aid management.
5. Explain Heimlich Maneuver stepwise.

6.2: EMERGENCY RESUSCITATION

CHAPTER OUTLINE

- Victim Assessment: Airway, Breathing, Circulation
- Airway Obstruction
- Basic Life Support (CPR)

INTRODUCTION

If the brain is deprived of oxygen for 4 minutes irreversible changes take place in it. The aim of respiratory resuscitation is the immediate oxygenation of the blood in order to forestall such changes. The urgent need for oxygenated blood is such that the lungs should be inflated, if possible even before attempting to remove debris from the mouth or air passage.

VICTIM ASSESSMENT

The first aider can assess the victim for injuries and surrounding environment once they have confirmed that they are breathing and have a strong pulse. Whether the victim is conscious or not, the evaluation should go as follows:

- **Scene safety:** Carefully approach the patient, ensuring that neither you nor any onlookers are in risk. Be mindful of any risks from gas, electricity, etc.
- **Patient assessment:** Carefully shake the patient's shoulder and call out: "Hello can you hear me?" **(Fig. 6.2.1)**. Continue the steps given in **Table 6.2.1**.

Opening the Airway (Fig. 6.2.2)

- Clear the airway by applying chin lift position.
- Ascertain that the patient is lying on his back; if required, roll him over.
- Lean his head back and place one hand on his forehead.
- Your second hand's fingers should be placed along the jawline.
- Utilizing the fingers, raise the chin.
- The "head tilt chin raise" combination of moves will open the airway.

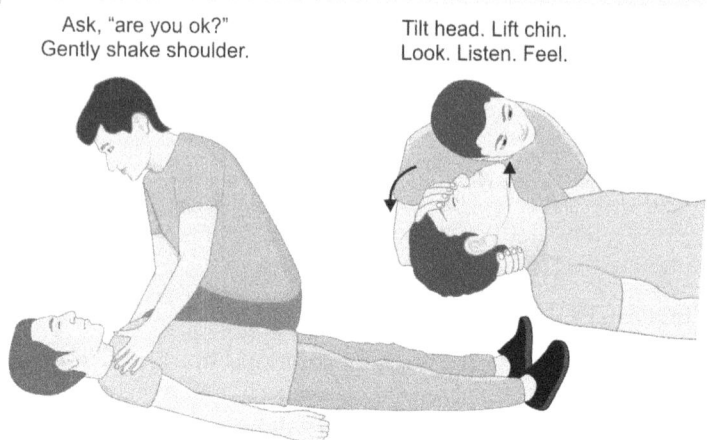

Fig. 6.2.1: Assessment of victim.

Table 6.2.1: Victim assessment.

Victim responds	Victim is unresponsive
• Provided there is no more threat, leave the victim in the position where you found him • Attempt to determine what the victim's issue is • If required, call for help • Regularly reassess the victim	Assess for Airway, Breathing and circulation

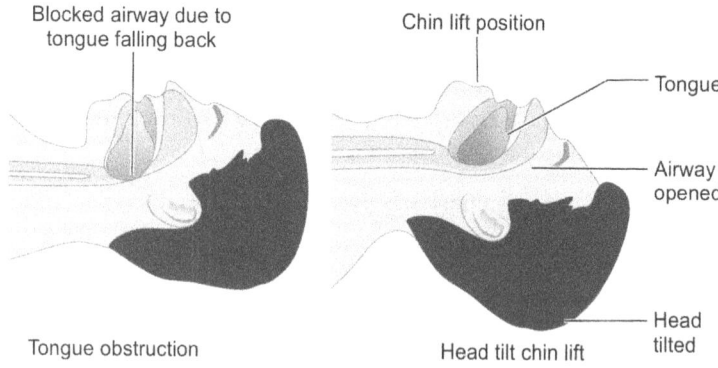

Fig. 6.2.2: Airway obstruction assessment.

❖ After the patient begins to breathe, place him or her in the recovery position.

Check for Breathing

- While keeping the airway open, check whether the patient is breathing normally.
- Look, listen and feel for any sign of respiration.

> **Look:** Rise and fall of chest.
> **Listen:** Assume the airway is not entirely open if the casualty's chest doesn't rise. Reposition your head and jaw, then look at yourself.
> **Feel:** Air coming out of the nose or mouth.
> See **Figure 6.2.1.**

Check for Circulation (Fig. 6.2.3)

- Check for presence of pulse in the neck (carotid pulse).
- Place two fingertips on the voice box of victim and slide them down into the space between the voice box and the nearby muscle to feel this pulse.
- Patient is placed in supine position and has their trunk slightly elevated when the carotid arterial pulses are being assessed.

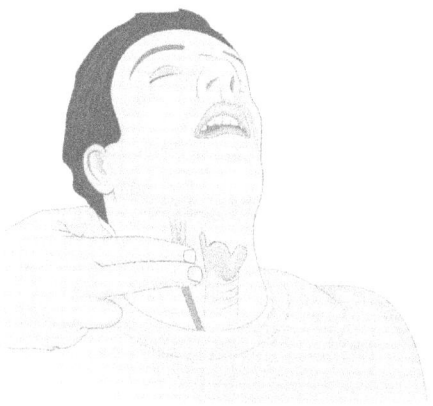

Fig. 6.2.3: Check circulation (carotid pulse).

AIRWAY OBSTRUCTION

Foreign body airway obstruction (FBAO) is one of the more common life-threatening emergencies that is seen and can be treated by common man.

General Guidelines

- For the purpose of clearing FBAO in cognizant infants younger than 1 year olds, a combination of back strikes and chest compression should be performed.
- Abdominal thrusts, back blows, and chest thrust relieve FBAO in conscious adults and children >1 year.
- These procedures should be carried out quickly one after another until the obstruction is removed; many procedures may be required for adults and children older than one year who are cognizant.

Causes

- **Adults:** Food
- **Children:** Food, coins, toys

First Aid Measures

For Adults and Children >1 Year Old

First aid management of FBAO depends on the types of obstruction whether it is mild or severe. It is important to ask the conscious victim "Are you choking?" Stepwise management is already discussed in Management of Choking given in Chapter 6.1.

For Infants (≤1 Year Old) (Fig. 6.2.4)

Mild airway obstruction	Complete airway obstruction (Conscious)
• Continue to observe the infant for development of severe airway obstruction. Do nothing else. • A chest compression and back blows during aggressive therapy could aggravate the airway blockage and result in potentially serious consequences.	• With the head lower than the torso, place the newborn face down along your arm. • Support the child in a head-down, prone position so that gravity can help with the foreign body removal. • The rescuer should seat or on their knees to safely support the infant over their lap. • Place the thumb of one hand at the angle of the lower jaw, and one or two fingers from the same hand at the same position on the other side of the jaw, to support the infant's head. • Keep your chin's soft tissues from being compressed. • With the heel of your other hand, strike the victim up to five times (back blow) between the shoulder blades. • Make that the airway obstruction has been relieved after each back blow.

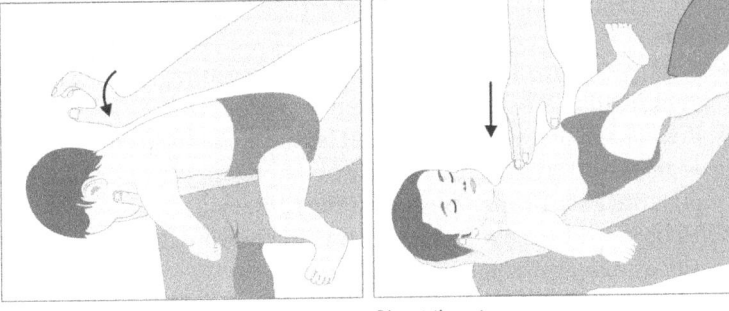

Back blows   Chest thrusts

Fig. 6.2.4: Airway obstruction first aid.

If five back blows fail to relieve the airway obstruction, give up to five chest thrusts as follows:
1. Position the child in a supine, head-down position.
2. To do this safely, place the free arm behind the infant's back and wrap the hand around the back of the head.
3. Support the child with your arm as it is resting against (or across) your thigh.
4. Give chest thrusts (compress approximately 1/3 of the depth of the chest).
5. Repeat up to five times.
6. Continue alternating five chest thrusts with five back blows if the impediment is still present.

If the victim becomes unconscious or is found unconscious:
1. Support the victim while you gently lower them to a solid surface.
2. Immediately contact for medical assistance if it hasn't already shown up or been requested.
3. Open the airway.
4. Breathe two to five times to help. If a breath during the initial attempts at rescue breathing does not cause the chest to rise, adjust the position of the head before trying again.
5. Start the compression phase of the cardiopulmonary resuscitation (CPR) protocol.

BASIC LIFE SUPPORT (RESUSCITATION)

CPR is an emergency procedure which is performed in an effort to manually preserve intact brain function until further measures are

taken to restore spontaneous blood circulation and breathing in a person.
- Compression/circulation, airway, breathing (C-A-B) and defibrillation are the accurate steps to be followed.
- Press down on the sternum for at least 2 inches (5-6 cm) at a rate of at least 100 per minute (nearly 2 compressions per second) but no more than 120 per minute during CPR.
- To begin CPR on a drowning victim, the priority should be upper airway management and rescue breaths.
- Cardiopulmonary resuscitation (CPR) should begin immediately if the victim is not breathing normally, or unconscious (unresponsive).

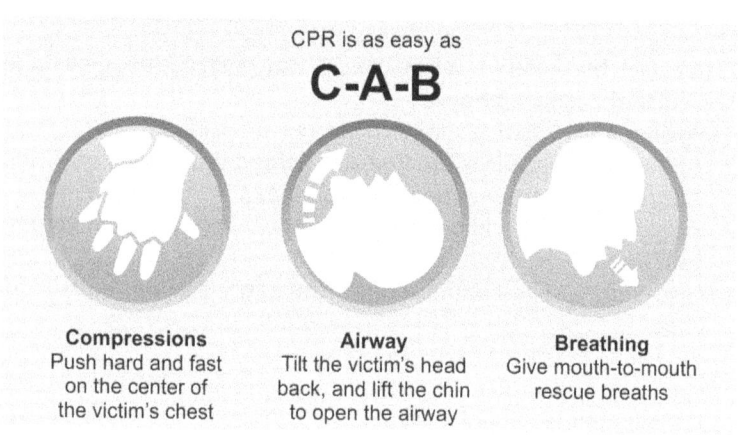

Steps in CPR

- Thumping the heart region.
- External cardiac compression.
- Mouth to mouth respiration.
  - **Two rescuers:** One rescuer perform emergency cardiovascular care (ECC) 30 times followed by the other rescuer performing mouth to mouth respiration twice, repeat.
  - **Single rescuer:** Emergency cardiovascular care (ECC) 30 times followed by mouth-to-mouth respiration twice—given by the same person.
  - If you are not able, or willing to give rescue breaths, perform compression-only CPR. Compression only CPR will maintain blood flow to the brain and has proven to be effective.

Guidelines in CPR

- Compression only CPR should be used by untrained or minimally trained first aid responders treating an adult victim.
- Compressions with breaths should be used by formally trained first responders (and professionals) treating an adult victim.
- Every effort should be made to reduce the time until compressions and to minimize any compression interruptions.
- The preferred method of CPR for infants and children with cardiac arrest is compressions with breaths.
- For infants, children and drowning victims who are unresponsive and not breathing, breaths should be given before compressions (Either two or five breaths may be given).
- Professional rescuers may be taught to do a pulse check, but this should not increase assessment time and is preferred to be done with the breathing check.
- Professional rescuers should check for pulse and if unsure as to whether the pulse is present, they should act as if the pulse is absent.
- For adults, the compression rate may be at least 100 per minute and not exceed 120 compressions per minute.
- For adults, the depth of compression may be at least 2 inches (5-6 cm).

Application of CPR

For the Unconscious Victim

- The initial action is to make sure that one-self, other first aiders, the victim and any bystanders are safe.
- Assess victim response by gently shaking his or her shoulders and asking loudly: "Are you all right?"

If the Victim Responds

- Do not move the victim.
- Assess the victim and if there is no further danger, leave the victim in the position in which you found him or her.
- Try to determine what is wrong with the victim and call for help if needed.
- Reassess the victim regularly.

If the Victim Does Not Respond

Shout for help, turn the victim onto his or her back.
- Open the airway using head tilt and chin lift.

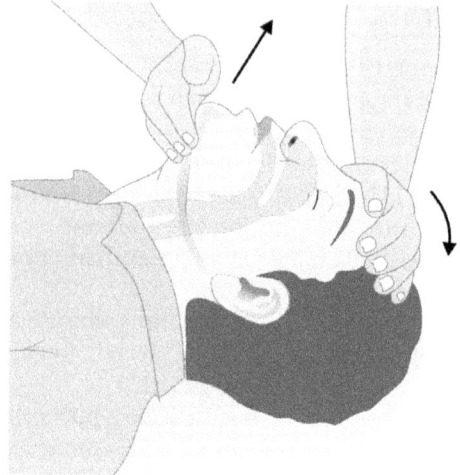

Fig. 6.2.5: Chin lift to open airway.

- Keep your thumb and index finger free to close the victim's nose if rescue breathing is required.
- With your fingertips under the point of the victim's chin, lift the chin to open the airway (**Figure 6.2.5**).
- Keeping the airway open, look, listen and feel for normal breathing.
- Look for chest and/or abdominal movement and listen to the victim's mouth for breath sounds or feel for air on your cheek.
- In case of professional rescuers', check for pulse simultaneously.

> **Note:**
> - Victim might be barely breathing or taking infrequent noisy gaps. Do not confused this with normal breathing.
> - Look, listen and feel for a maximum of 10 seconds.
> - Even if there is a slight doubt whether breathing is present, then assume it is not.

If the Victim is Breathing

- If there is a suspected cervical spine injury, place the patient in recovery position (**Figure 6.2.6**).
- Send/go for help.
- Reassess continuously whether the victim is breathing normally.

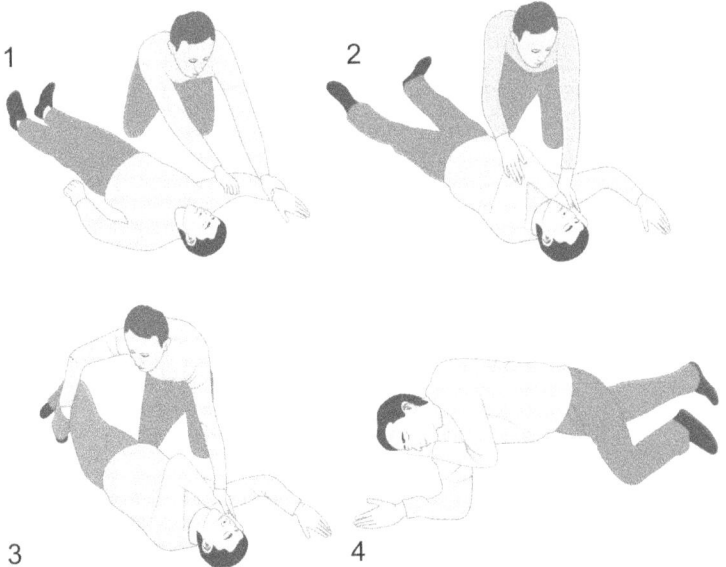

Fig. 6.2.6: Placing victim in recovery position.

If the victim is not breathing (for lay rescuers and with no pulse for professional rescuers
- Shout or send someone for help.
- Kneel by the victim side and start chest compression **(Fig. 6.2.7)**.
- Place the heel of one hand in the centre of the victim's chest and place the heel of your other hand on top of the first hand.
- Ensure that pressure is not applied over the victim's ribs.
- Do not exert any pressure over the upper abdomen or the bottom end of bony sternum's (breastbone).
- With your arms straight and in a vertical position above the victim's chest **(Fig. 6.2.8)**, press down on the sternum at a rate of at least 100 compressions per minute (almost 2 compressions per second), but no more than 120 compressions per minute.
- Release all of the pressure on the chest after each compression without letting go of your grip on the sternum; compression and release should be equally timed.

SECTION 2: First Aid Management

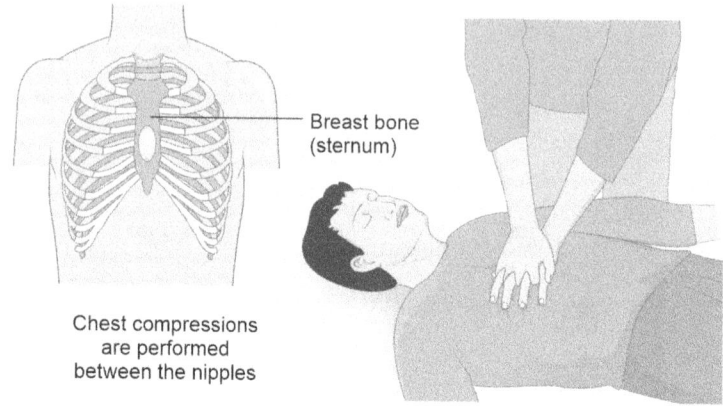

Fig. 6.2.7: Correct position for chest compression.

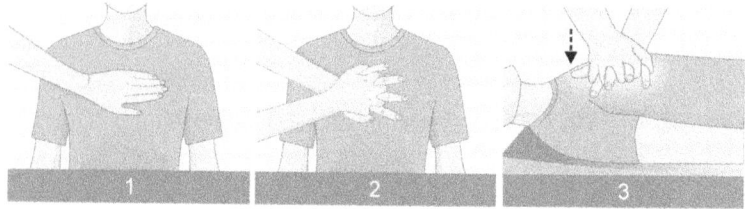

Fig. 6.2.8: Proper technique of hand placement for chest compression.

Chest Compression with Rescue Breaths

- Open the airway again using head tilt and chin lift, after 30 compressions.
- Using the index finger and thumb of the hand that is on the victim forehead, pinch the soft part of the victim's nose closed.
- Maintain chin lift but allow the mouth to open.
- Take a regular breath and make sure you have a good seal, blow steadily into the victim's mouth while keeping an eye out for the victim's chest to rise.
- Maintaining head tilt and chin lift, take your mouth away from the victim and watch for the chest to fall as air passes out.
- Take another normal breath and blow into the victim's mouth once more, for a total of two effective rescue breaths.'
- Before returning to chest compressions, do not attempt to take more than two breaths at a time. Give 30 extra chest compressions

to the person as soon as you place your hands back in the proper location on their chest. Make a loud count.
- ❖ Maintain a 30:2 ratio of chest compression with rescue breaths.

> **Note:**
> Before trying again, make sure the victim's mouth is clear of any obstruction and that there is an adequate head tilt and chin lift (as described in Chapter 2). This is because if your initial rescue breath does not cause the victim's chest to rise as in normal breathing, the obstruction may be in the victim's mouth. To avoid becoming fatigued, if there are multiple rescuers available, they should alternate performing CPR every 1-2 minutes. Make sure that chest compressions continue when the rescuers switch over.

For Compression-only CPR

- ❖ Only perform chest compressions if you are unable or unwilling to perform rescue breathing.
- ❖ If only chest compressions are administered, they must be done continuously and at a minimum rate of 100 per minute.
- ❖ Only if the victim obviously wakes up and starts moving around should you decide to stop resuscitating them. If not, continue.
- ❖ Maintain uninterrupted resuscitation until professional medical assistance comes and assumes control or the victim begins to breathe properly.

If the victim is not breathing and has a pulse (for professional rescuers)

- ❖ Send someone for help.
- ❖ Kneel by the victim's side.
- ❖ Using your index finger and thumb from the hand that is on the victim's forehead, try pinching the soft section of the victim's nose closed.
- ❖ Open the mouth but keep the chin upward.
- ❖ This is a good rescue breath. Take a regular breath and make sure you have a good seal, blow steadily into the victim's mouth while keeping an eye out for the victim's chest to rise.
- ❖ Maintaining head tilt and chin lift, take your mouth away from the victim and watch for the chest to fall as air passes out.
- ❖ Continue delivering breaths at a rate of 1 breath per 5 seconds.
- ❖ Periodically recheck for pulse and if the victim begins to breathe and/or move around, perform a complete reassessment.

SECTION 2: First Aid Management

Note
If your initial rescue breath does not make the victim's chest rise as in normal breathing, then before your next attempt, provide care of a foreign body airway obstruction.

Resuscitation of children after recognizing a cardiac arrest (a victim that is unresponsive and not breathing), first aid providers should perform the following:

- Prior to beginning of chest compressions, provide 2 to 5 first rescue breaths. This is a good rescue breath. Take a regular breath and make sure you have a good seal, blow steadily into the victim's mouth while keeping an eye out for the victim's chest to rise.
- Take your mouth off the victim while maintaining the victim's head tilt and chin lift and watch for the chest to drop as air escapes.
- If you're the only rescuer, give CPR for about a minute before calling for assistance. Reduce the chest's volume by about one-third of its depth.
- While compressing a child <1 year of age, use two fingers **(Fig. 6.2.9)**; when compressing a child >1 year of age, use one or both hands, depending on the situation.
- Continue to do 30 compressions, then two breaths (30:2).

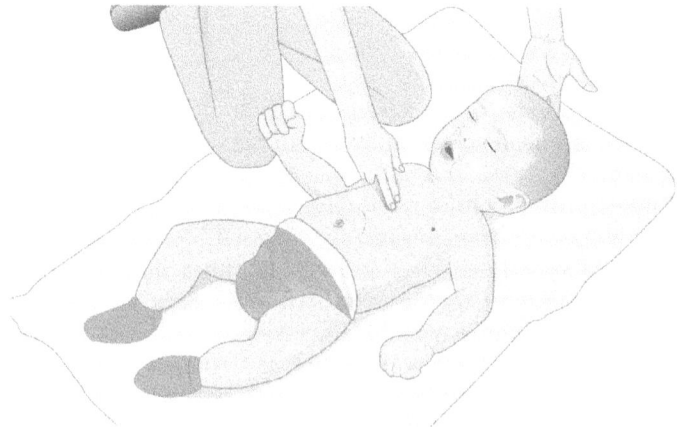

Fig. 6.2.9: CPR of infant.

Note:
Rechecking the victim should only be delayed until the patient is visibly awake and moving around; otherwise, do not stop CPR. If there are multiple rescuers on the scene, they should alternate performing CPR every one to two minutes to avoid getting tired and using a ratio of 15 compressions to 2 breaths. Make sure that chest compressions continue when the rescuers switch over. The same actions—five first breaths and one minute of CPR performed by a lone rescuer—could enhance the outcomes for drowning victims. Only people with a specific duty of care for prospective drowning victims or trained rescuers should be taught this modified version of CPR (e.g., lifeguards).

REVIEW QUESTIONS

LONG ESSAYS

1. Define emergency resuscitation. Describe the various methods of victim assessment.
2. Explain the steps applied in the management of airway obstruction in infants.
3. Describe steps of performing CPR in adults.

SHORT ESSAYS

1. Explain chest thrust methods.
2. Guidelines of CPR.
3. Explain C-A-B.
4. Methods for application of CPR in children.
5. Explain chest compression with Rescue breaths.

Unconsciousness 7

CHAPTER OUTLINE

- Common Cause of Unconsciousness
- Direct Injury to the Brain
- Apoplexy
- Epilepsy
- Hysteria
- Infantile Convulsions
- Effects of Excessive Heat
- Diabetes and Insulin Overdose
- Fainting
- Heart Attacks

INTRODUCTION

Consciousness is the awareness of oneself and the environment and the ability to respond to external stimuli. Unconsciousness (insensibility) is loss of consciousness (LOC) due to interruption of the action of the brain through some interference with the functions of the nervous system. It is an important indication not only of disease or of injury to the brain, but of many serious injuries or diseases of other parts of the body. There are two degrees of unconsciousness apart from sleep:
1. Partial (stupor).
2. Complete (coma).

The degree of unconsciousness may be determined by the following:

- **Check for responsiveness:** Carefully shake the patients shoulder and shouts: "Hello can you hear me?"
- In Stupor he/she can be roused with difficulty varying with the degree of stupor present. In coma there is no response.
- In stupor the casualty objects to the eyelashes being touched or resists attempt to draw back the eyelids. This is shown by twitching or contraction of the eyelids. In coma there is no response.
- Response of the pupils of the eyes to light.

The pupil of the eye is the dark circle surrounded by a colored muscular ring (iris). In the normal person a bright light falling on the eye causes the iris to contract and the size of the pupil is diminished.

In the dark, the iris relaxes, and the pupil dilates. If a bright light is flashed into the eyes or if the eyes are shaded and the shade is suddenly removed, the pupils become smaller in stupor, but remain fixed in deep coma. This reaction may vary with the degree of stupor present. In deep coma the pupils are often widely dilated.

COMMON CAUSES OF UNCONSCIOUSNESS

Common causes of unconsciousness include a large number of medical and surgical diseases such as inflammation of the brain, etc. The diagnosis of these is beyond the scope of the first aider, but intelligent application of the 'general rules for the treatment of an unconscious person' will enable him/her to render first aid in all cases. In some cases of unconsciousness convulsions are present. There are spasmodic and involuntary contractions of the muscles of the body and limbs. They may be general, affecting the whole of the body or they may be limited to the limbs or one side of the body. A convulsion is commonly known as a fits. Some common causes are listed below:

- Anaphylactic shock (*refer* Chapter 3.3)
- Shock (*refer* Chapter 3.3)
- Asphyxia (*refer* Chapter 6.1)
- Poisoning (*refer* Chapter 10.1)
- Head injury associated with injury to the brain causing concussion or compression
- Apoplexy
- Epilepsy
- Hysteria
- Infantile convulsions
- Effects of excessive heat
- Diabetes and insulin overdose
- Fainting
- Heart attacks

GENERAL RULES FOR MANAGEMENT OF AN UNCONSCIOUS PERSON
- Ensure an abundant supply of fresh air and the air passages are not obstructed:
  - Remove from harmful gases or impure atmosphere.
  - Open windows and doors.
  - Keep crowds at bay.
  - Remove dentures, if present.
- If breathing has stopped or appears to be failing, turn the casualty into prone position and commence artificial respiration.

- If breathing is not noisy lay the casualty on his/her back with the head and shoulders slightly raised and support, and turn the head to one side. Be prepared to modify the position if breathing becomes difficult or obstructed.
- If breathing is noisy (bubbling through secretions) turn the casualty into the three-quarter prone position. Support him/her in this position with a pad in front of the chest or draw up the upper knee. If the casualty is on a stretcher, raise the feet of the stretcher to help to drain secretions from the lungs.
- Undo all tight clothing about the neck, chest and waist.
- Apply the special treatment for the condition that has caused the unconsciousness.
- Wrap in a blanket, but do not apply heat.
- Do not leave the casualty until he/she has been placed in the charge of a responsible person. Keep a continuous and careful watch for any change in casualty condition.
- Do not attempt to give food or fluids, while the casualty is unconscious.
- Shift him/her to shelter as a stretcher case as soon as possible.
- When he/she returns to consciousness moisten the lips with water. Unless an abdominal injury is suspected, sips of water may be given if complains of thirst.

Direct Injury to the Brain

Direct injury to the brain may bring out either concussion or compression.

Compression

Compression is a condition due to actual pressure on same part of the brain within the skull by blood clot or a piece of bone as in fracture of the skull. It may follow concussion with no return to consciousness or may come on after apparent recovery. During the early stages of compression signs of irritation of the brain may occur. There are twitching of the limbs, crying out or shouting or even convulsions. The first aider should be prepared for this to happen in cases of head injury. The casualty should not be forcibly restrained but protected from injuring himself/herself.

Signs and Symptoms

Most all of the following signs will usually be present, but the absence of some or any of them does not rule out a diagnosis of compression:
- **Unconsciousness:** Coma may be present, or its onset may be delayed or it may follow a period of stupor.
- Face is flushed.

- Breathing is noisy.
- Pulse is slow.
- Body temperature may be raised. The head may feel hot to touch.
- Pupils of the eyes may be unequal in size, or they may be dilated.
- Paralysis on one side of the body may be present.

First Aid Measures
- Apply the general rules for the treatment of unconsciousness.
- Compression is a serious condition and medical aid must be obtained as soon as possible.

Concussion (Fig. 7.1)
Concussion is a condition of widespread disturbance of the functions of the brain, which comes on as a result of injury to the head and sometimes to the spine. It is not necessarily associated with any changes in the brain substance. A blow on the head, a fall from a height or to the feet or the buttocks, or a blow on the point of the jaw may all cause concussion, by jarring through the base of the skull.

First Aid Measures
- Apply the general rules for management of unconscious patient.
- Avoid unnecessary movements.

(The symptoms and first aid measures for concussion is Chapter 4.2.)

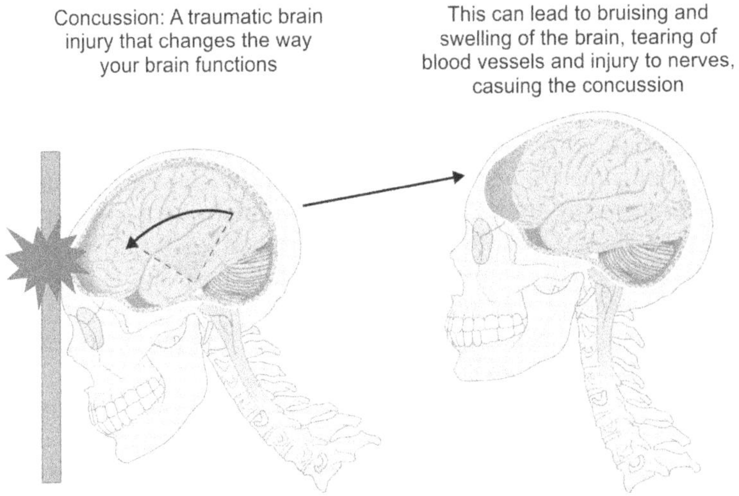

Concussion: A traumatic brain injury that changes the way your brain functions

This can lead to bruising and swelling of the brain, tearing of blood vessels and injury to nerves, casuing the concussion

Fig. 7.1: Concussion.

Apoplexy

Apoplexy occurs most commonly in middle aged or elderly people with high blood pressure. It is due to the rupture of a diseased blood vessel causing hemorrhage into the brain tissue or to a clot of blood interfering with the blood supply to part of the brain. It is commonly called 'stroke'.

Signs and Symptoms

Signs and symptoms are similar to compression. The age of the casualty, the sudden onset and the absence of history or signs of injury help with the diagnosis.

Treatment

Apply the general rules for the treatment of unconsciousness.

Epilepsy

Epilepsy is a condition which may occur at any age, but usually first appears in young persons. Persons with epilepsy are liable to recurrent attacks, which may be of two types—minor and major.

Types

- **Minor epilepsy:** The casualty may become pale with eyes fixed and staring and may become momentarily unconscious. He/she may then resume his/her previous activity as though nothing has occurred. The above-mentioned condition will lost for few seconds, may reoccur in a day several times.
- **Major epilepsy:** The casualty may have a premonition that he/she is going to have a fits. He/she may experience a sense of strangeness accompanied by headache, irritability, restlessness or a feeling of lethargy—the 'dreamy state'. These sensations are known as the 'aura'. The epileptic fits consist of four stages:
  1. The casualty suddenly loses consciousness and falls to the ground, possibly with a cry.
  2. He/she remains rigid for some seconds and during this stage the face becomes flushed or even livid.
  3. The convulsions start, and the casualty may injure himself/herself by striking a hard object. He/she froths at the mouth and may bite his/her tongue. He/she will not have control of his/her bladder or bowel and may pass urine and motions involuntarily (incontinence).

4. After a variable time, usually a few minutes, the convulsions cease, and the casualty may be dazed and confused or sometimes act in a strange manner without realizing what He/she is doing. This is called post-epileptic automatism. This condition lasts for a few hours to few days.

Treatment

- Restrain the casualty only so far, as is necessary. Forcible restraints of an epileptic may cause injury. If possible, remove any objects against which he/she might injure himself/herself.
- Loosen tight clothing, roll a cloth or sweater/shirt and place it under the casualty head to prevent head injury **(Fig. 7.2)**.
- As opportunity arises place the handle of a spoon or other hard object wrapped in a handkerchief between his/her teeth to prevent the casualty from biting his/her tongue.
- Wipe away the froth from his/her mouth.
- Apply the general rules for the treatment of unconsciousness.
- Keep a careful watch for a possible recurrence and do not leave him/her until one is satisfied that he/she is fully aware of his/her surroundings or until he/she is placed in the care of another responsible person.
- Advice the casualty to see his/her doctor.

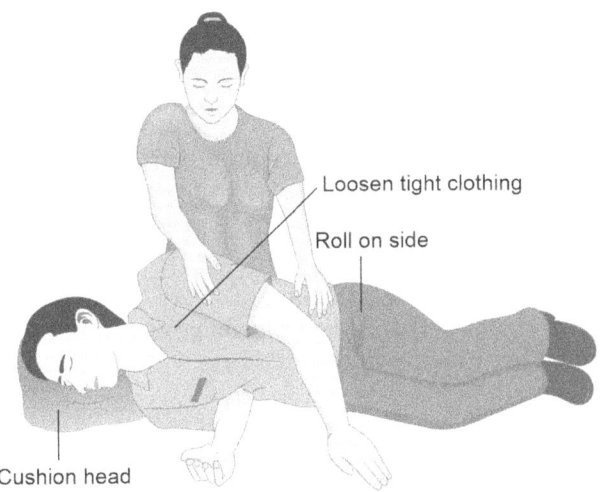

Fig. 7.2: First aid for epilepsy.

Hysterical Fits

Hysterical attacks occurs most frequently in persons of 'nervous disposition'. They are said to be more common in women, but men are also subject to them. The usual cause is an emotional crisis or mental stress.

Signs and Symptoms

Signs and symptoms vary from a temporary loss of emotional control to more serious signs including rigidity of the body and apparent convulsions. The 'Hysterical convulsions may appear in a dramatic manner demanding an audience and does not occur, therefore, when the casualty is alone the following conditions may occur:

- The casualty may fall, taking care not to injure himself/herself.
- He/she may laugh, cry or utter words.
- The 'convulsions' consist of voluntary through purposeless movements such as tearing the hair or clutching at bystanders or rolling on the ground. There is never complete unconsciousness.

There may be occasions when there is doubt as to the diagnosis and the first aider must be guided by the general circumstances and facts before deciding to treat the condition as or a hysterical attack.

Treatment

- If the first aider after careful consideration of all the circumstances is satisfied that he/she is dealing with a hysterical attack, he/she should not show too much sympathy or concern.
- He/she should speak firmly to the casualty but should not bully or threaten.
- The casualty should be kept under observation until he/she has recovered sufficiently control of himself/herself and then be given something to do.

Infantile Convulsions

Infantile convulsions occur in infants as a result of teething, some stomach or chest trouble or when sickening for an illness such as an infectious disease may be due to high fever.

Signs and Symptoms

- General twitching or tremor of the muscles.
- Extreme pallor and later blueness of the face.
- Occasional squinting or upturned eyes.

- ❖ Holding of the breath.
- ❖ Froth may appear at the mouth.

Treatment

- ❖ Apply the general rules for the treatment of unconsciousness.
- ❖ Wrap the child in warm blankets.

> **Note:**
> If the child is having fits due to high fever, wrap the child in a wet cloth for 10–15 minutes and bring down the temperature and control the fits, later refer to the near doctor's clinic.

Effects of Excessive Heat

Heat exhaustion and heatstroke conditions arise from similar causes but vary considerably in their progress and treatment. Exposure to excessive heat, especially of a moist character, with or without physical exertion, conditions where the air and surroundings are hotter than the body, and it is difficult to get rid of heat from the body by the evaporation of sweat. Lack of fluids and salt are contributory causes. Exposure to excessive heat can cause dizziness and fainting. Effects of heat and its first aid measures will be discussed further in Chapter 11.

Diabetic Coma and Insulin Overdose (Insulin Coma/Insulin Shock)

Diabetic coma can occur due to severe high blood sugar or low blood sugar levels, it is considered as a life-threatening condition that causes unconsciousness.

Signs and Symptoms of Diabetic Coma and Insulin Overdose (Table 7.1)

Table 7.1: Signs of diabetic and insulin coma.

Diabetic coma	Insulin overdose
Dry skin	Skin is moist with respiration
Sigh and deep breathing	Breathing is shallow and quiet
Breath may smell of acetone (musty apple or nail varnish)	Breath is odorless, there may be excitability.
There may be varying degrees of unconsciousness	Faintness or unconsciousness may be present

Treatment

- Apply the general rules for the treatment of unconsciousness.
- Get a doctor immediately or if this is not possible admit to hospital.
- In insulin overdose: If the casualty can swallow:
  - Feed with sweet substances, dissolved sugar, jam or sweets given with a teaspoon.
  - Ability to swallow may be tested by putting a teaspoon full of cold water between the gums and the cheek.

Fainting

A faint is a brief loss of consciousness of no more than momentary duration caused by a temporary reduction in the flow of blood to the brain. Recovery is usually rapid and complete.

It may be a nervous reaction to pain or fright, or the result of an emotional upset, exhaustion or lack of food. It is, however, more common after long periods of physical inactivity, especially in warm atmosphere, where lack of muscular activity causes a large volume of blood to collect in the lower part of the body and legs. This reduces the amount of blood available to the circulation, e.g., as in a soldier standing on parade.

Signs and Symptoms

- Pulse will be slow at first (this is an important clue) and weak
- Casualty may be very pale
- The skin is cold and clammy
- The breathing is shallow.

First Aid Measures

Aim: Position the casualty, so that gravity helps to increase the flow of blood to the brain.

Prevention

- If the casualty is on parade or standing in a crowd, advise him/her to flex the leg muscles and toes to aid circulation.
- If the casualty feels unsteady, make to sit down and help to lean forward with his/her head between the knees and advise to take deep breaths as shown in **Figure 7.3A**.

Treatment

- When a casualty faints, lay him/her down with legs raised and maintain an open airway **(Fig. 7.3 B)**.

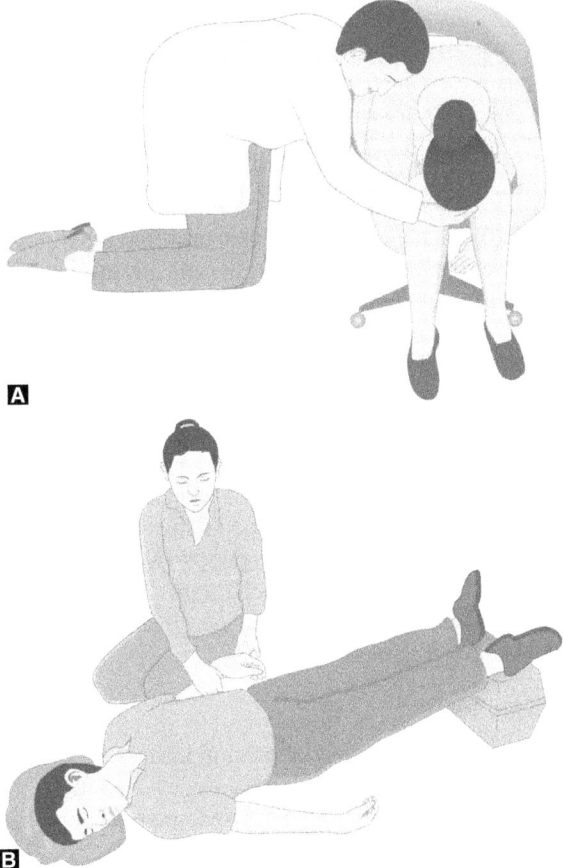

Figs. 7.3A and B: (A) Prevention measure for fainting; (B) Leg elevation.

- Loosen any tight clothing at his/her neck, chest and waist, to assist circulation and breathing.
- Make sure that the casualty has plenty of fresh air; place in a current of fresh air and fan air on his/her face. If necessary, place in the shade.
- Reassure whilst, if he/she is regaining consciousness; gradually raise his/her to a sitting position.
- Check for and treat any injury that he/she may have sustained on falling.
- Check breathing rate, pulse and level of responsiveness until fully recovered.

> **Note:**
> ‹‹ Do not give the casualty anything by mouth until he/she is fully conscious.
> ‹‹ Do not give to the casualty any alcohol.

Stroke

The term 'stroke' is used to describe a condition in which the blood supply to part of the brain is suddenly or critically impaired by a blood clot (cerebral thrombosis) or when a ruptured artery leaks blood into the brain (cerebral hemorrhage). The latter is more likely in people who have high blood pressure. In either case, the affected brain cells cease to function altogether.

Each area of the brain controls a different system or part of the body, and any deficiency resulting from a stroke depends on how much and which part of the brain is affected. Major strokes are often fatal, but many people make successful recoveries from minor strokes. Strokes are more common in people over 55, in those who are known to suffer from blackouts or circulatory disorders or in those who have had previous strokes. The symptoms and signs may be confused with drunkenness.

Signs and Symptoms

- Possible sudden severe headache or giddiness.
- A strong pulse.
- Casualty may be disoriented, confused, anxious or weeping.
- Progressive loss of consciousness.
- Depending on the extent of the stroke one or more of the following physical defects may be also apparent.
- Paralysis of mouth: The corner of the mouth may droop, saliva may dribble from it, and speech may be slurred.
- Weakness and decreased sensation in one or both limbs and on one side of the body.
- Flushed face with hot dry skin.
- Pupils may be unequal.
- Loss of bladder and bowel control.

First Aid Measures

Aim: Minimize the effects of damage to the brain and arrange immediate admission in the hospital.

Treatment

- If the casualty is conscious, lay him/her down with head and shoulders slightly raised and supported. Position his/her head on the side to allow saliva to drain from the mouth.
- Loosen any constricting clothing around neck, chest and waist to assist circulation and breathing.

Note
Do not give the casualty anything by mouth.

- If the casualty becomes unconscious, open his/her airway and check breathing. Complete the C-A-B of resuscitation, if required and place him/her in the recovery position.
- Arrange urgent transportation to hospital. Transport as a stretcher case maintaining the treatment position.

REVIEW QUESTIONS

LONG ESSAYS

1. List the common cause of unconsciousness and explain epilepsy and its first aid management.
2. Describe stroke in details.
3. Explain unconsciousness due to head injury.

SHORT ESSAYS

1. First aid measures for fainting.
2. Signs of diabetic coma and insulin overdose.
3. Apoplexy.
4. Infantile convulsions.
5. Hysterical fits.

Foreign Bodies 8

CHAPTER OUTLINE

- Splinters
- Foreign Body in the Eye
- Foreign Body in the Nose
- Foreign Body in the Throat
- Foreign Body in the Stomach

INTRODUCTION

A 'foreign body' means any extraneous matter that enters the body either through a wound in the skin (penetrating) or via one of the natural openings of the body (inserted or swallowed), or that enters the eye. A penetrating foreign body can be anything that enters the body, from a tiny splinter of wood or glass to a large wooden stake or piece of metal. It may be loose and easily removed without causing further pain or injury or it can be embedded in the skin. The latter may in addition, be acting as a plug preventing blood loss. Large embedded foreign bodies may produce a deep wound, but small splinters cause little more than minor lacerations. The main problem with injuries involving penetrating foreign bodies is that foreign bodies are rarely clean so there is a high risk of infection.

SPLINTERS

Wood and metal splinters, which have become embedded in the skin, are probably the most common foreign bodies **(Fig. 8.1A)**. They can generally be removed with tweezers **(Fig. 8.1B)**. However, if the splinter is deeply embedded or over a joint, seek medical aid as soon as possible.

Signs and Symptoms

- Known contact with pieces of wood, metal or glass.

CHAPTER 8: Foreign Bodies

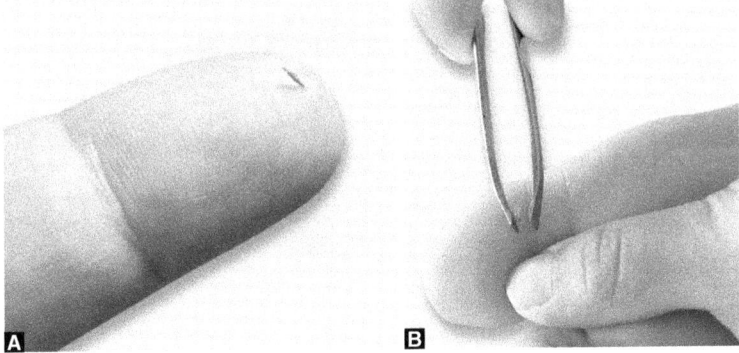

Figs. 8.1A and B: (A) Wood splinters embedded in skin; (B) Removing the splinter out using a sterilize tweezers.

- An embedded foreign body may be visible.
- Pain and tenderness in the area.

First Aid Measures

Aim: To gently remove the splinters out.
- If the area around the splinter is dirty, cleanse it using soap and water.
- Sterilize a pair of tweezers by passing them through flame.
- Gently try to pull the splinter out of the wound with tweezers. Hold the tweezers as near to the skin as possible and grasp the splinter. Pull the splinter out in the opposite directions to that in which it entered the skin.
- If the splinter does not come out easily or begins to break up, treat as an embedded foreign body and seek medical aid.

> **Note:**
> Do not probe the area to reach the splinter. Make sure the casualty's tetanus inoculation probe is up-to-date.

FOREIGN BODY IN THE EYE

Dust, grit, insects or loose eyelashes may get into the eye, causing great discomfort. If not quickly removed, they may cause serious trouble.

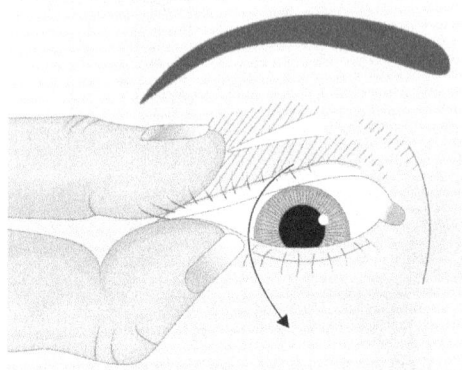

Fig. 8.2: Removing foreign body from eye.

First Aid Measures

- ❖ Avoid rubbing the eyes. Blink the eyes rapidly a few times. This may help to dislodge the foreign body.
- ❖ If it feels the foreign body is under the upper lid, grasp the lid by the lashes and pull it forward over the lower lid, then released it. This may dislodge the foreign body (**Fig. 8.2**).
- ❖ Another method is to flood the eye with clean water, e.g., by holding the nose and dipping the face into a basin of water, then bending.
- ❖ Try turning back the upper lid over a matchstick, while the casualty looks down. The foreign body is often found near to the edge of the lid. Remove it with the corner of a clean handkerchief or a moistened swabs tick.
- ❖ If the foreign body cannot get out easily, supply antibiotic eye ointments, cover the eye with a bandage and refer the casualty to a doctor.

FOREIGN BODY IN THE EAR

Children often put beads, peas or other small things into the ear or nose. Insect sometimes get into the ear.

First Aid Measures

- ❖ If it is sure that an insect is in the ear, it may be floated out by pouring oil or spirits into the ear (**Fig. 8.3**).

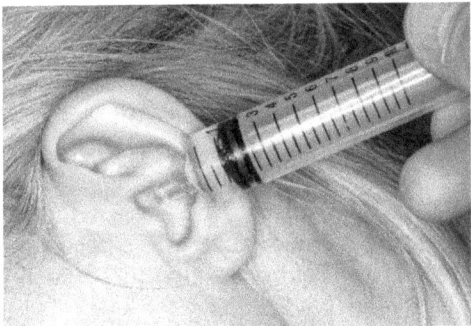

Fig. 8.3: Pouring oil in ear.

- All other foreign bodies must be left alone, and the casualty must be taken to a doctor. Because of the danger of pushing a foreign body further into the ear.

FOREIGN BODY IN THE NOSE

When this happens, one will be faced with a highly excited child who is both frightened and suffering from a sore nose. It is important therefore to show both tact and skill in dealing with this emergency.

First Aid Measures

- Take the history and establish how the accident happened and what the foreign body is.
- Calm the patient and reassure him/her in order to gain cooperation.
- Examine the nose to see how deep the foreign body has gone. If the foreign body is not too far in the nose, put thick wick made of cloth or take a feather.
- Try to tickle the unaffected nostril and make the child to sneeze as sneezing will help the foreign body in the nose to come out. If this fails, block the ears, mouth and normal nostrils with the fingers.
- Ask the patient to blow as hard as possible to dislodge the foreign body in the nose. If this also fails, take him/her to the nearby hospital and tell him/her to breathe through the mouth.
- Hold the child's hands, if necessary to prevent him/her doing harm to the nose.

FOREIGN BODY IN THE THROAT

First Aid Measures

- If the object stuck in the throat is small and harmless, give a glass of water to drink so that the object will probably pass on through the stomach and intestines without causing any harm.
- If an irregular and fairly big article is stuck in the throat, hold the child by the legs or lay him/her over knees, head downwards, then tap on the back of the neck or between the shoulders or the person can be made to vomit out the object.

Fishbone in the Throat

- If a fishbone or something sharp is caught in the throat, first aid measure is to spit out the food and cough forcefully to loosen the fishbone.
- Reassure the person and the relatives and refer to the health center or hospital at once.

FOREIGN BODY IN THE STOMACH

- When smooth objects such as seeds, coins or buttons are swallowed, they usually pass through the stomach and intestines out of the body. There is neither need for panic nor for any treatment. The case may be shown to a doctor.
- If a sharp or blunt objects such as glass pieces are swallowed, then patient should be taken to the nearest health center.

REVIEW QUESTIONS

LONG ESSAYS

1. Explain foreign body in the eyes and its first aid measures.
2. Describe foreign body in nose.
3. Describe foreign body in ear and throat.

SHORT ESSAYS

1. First aid measures for splinters embedded on skin.
2. First aid measures for foreign body in stomach.
3. First aid measures for foreign body in the ear.
4. Foreign body in the throat.
5. First aid measures for fishbone caught in the throat.

Burns and Scalds 9

CHAPTER OUTLINE

- Definition
- Burns
- Types of Burns
- Classification of Burns
- Assessment of Burns
- General Guidelines for Treatment of Burns and Scalds
- Dry Burns and Scalds
- Burns in the Mouth and Throat
- Chemical Burns in the Skin
- Chemical Burns in the Eye
- Electrical Burns
- Snow Blindness, Welder's Flash and Radiation

INTRODUCTION

Burns and scalds are damage to the skin caused by heat. The effects of burns and scalds are the same. There may be reddening of the skin or blister formation or destruction of the skin or destruction of the deeper tissues. Pain is very severe. There is immediate danger from shock, which may be severe and made worse by the intense pain and by loss of plasma into the burnt area. Later there is danger from septic infection. The dangers of a burn increase with its surface area (even if it is only superficial) and if one third or more of the skin area is involved, the patient may become dangerously ill. In small children and especially in infants even small burns should be regarded serious injuries and medical aid sought without delay.

DEFINITION

Burns

A burn is an injury caused by:
- Dry heat such as fire, a piece of hot metal or the sun.
- Contact with any object charged with a high tension electric current or by lightning.
- Friction for example, by contact with a revolving wheel (brush burn) or fast-moving rope or wire.

- Corrosive chemicals:
  - Acids, such as sulphuric, nitric, hydrochloric.
  - Alkalis, such as caustic soda, caustic potash, strong ammonia or quicklime.

Scalds

A scald is an injury caused by moist heat, such as boiling water, steam, hot oil or tar, improperly applied poultice.

BURNS

Types of Burns

Burns can be categorized according to the cause of the injury.

1. **Dry burns:** Flames, lighted cigarettes and hot electrical equipment such as irons are all common causes of dry burns. Fast moving objects rubbed against the skin produce dry friction burns. Alternatively, they may be caused by the skin rubbing against an object. The most common example of this is 'rope burn' **(Fig. 9.1A)**.
2. **Scalds:** Wet heat such as steam, hot water or fat produces scalds **(Fig. 9.1B)**.
3. **Cold burns:** Cold burns may result from contact with metals in freezing conditions **(Fig. 9.1C)**. Freezing agents such as liquid oxygen and liquid nitrogen can also cause cold burns.
4. **Chemical burns:** Acids and alkalis found in domestic cleaning products as well as in industry may cause burns, if in contact with the skin **(Fig. 9.1D)**.
5. **Electrical burns:** Electric currents and lightning generate heat causing burn in the skin and its underlying tissues **(Fig. 9.1E)**.
6. **Radiation burns (Fig. 9.1F):** Sunrays and light reflected from a bright surface (e.g., snow) can cause damage to the skin and eyes. Very rarely, radiation burns can be caused by overexposure to X-rays or radioactive substances.

Classification of Burns

Burns are classified according to the area and depth of the injury. Any casualty with burns covering an area greater than 2-3 cm (1 inch) diameter, or burns deeper than the surface of the skin or burns arising from electrical contact, must be referred to a doctor or hospital.

- **Area:** The area of a burn gives a rough guide as to whether or not a casualty is likely to suffer stock. The greater the area involved, the

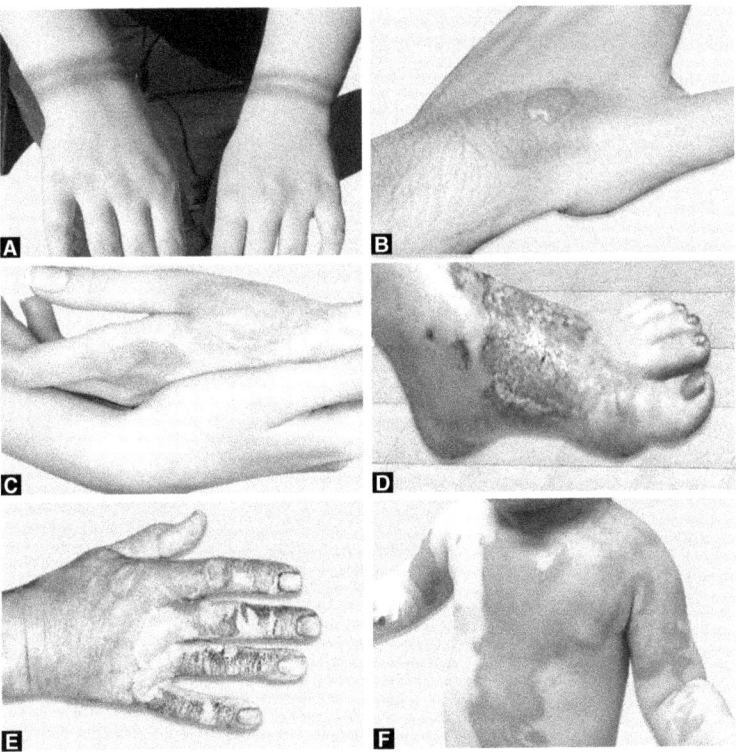

Figs. 9.1A to F: Types of burns: (A) Rope burn; (B) Scalds; (C) Cold burns; (D) Chemical burns; (E) Electrical burns; (F) Radiation burns.

greater the possibility of shock, because of greater fluid loss. For example, an adult casualty with a superficial burn covering 9% or more of the body's surface will need hospital treatment.
❖ **Depth of burns:** There are four levels of burning **(Table 9.1)**:
  1. Superficial.
  2. Superficial partial thickness.
  3. Deep partial thickness.
  4. Full thickness.

Assessment of Burns

The 'rule of nines' diagram **(Fig. 9.2)** divides the body surface into areas of 9%. Any injury of an equivalent area will require hospital

SECTION 2: First Aid Management

Table 9.1: Classification of burn wound (Vaughan and Beckel, 2012).

Burn wound	Derma layers involved	Wound characteristics	Healing
Superficial	Epidermis only	Redness, skin peeling, dry flaky skin	Heals in 3–5 days
Superficial-partial thickness	Epidermis, upper 1/3 Dermis	Painful blisters, edema, eschar formation	Heals in 1–2 weeks
Deep partial-thickness	Epidermis and all dermis	Red waxy white appearance, blisters, reduce pain formation, eschar formation	Heals in 2–3 weeks
Full thickness	Epidermis dermis, subcutaneous tissue	Bloodless pear-white, eschar formation, hair easily plucked.	Requires surgical intervention

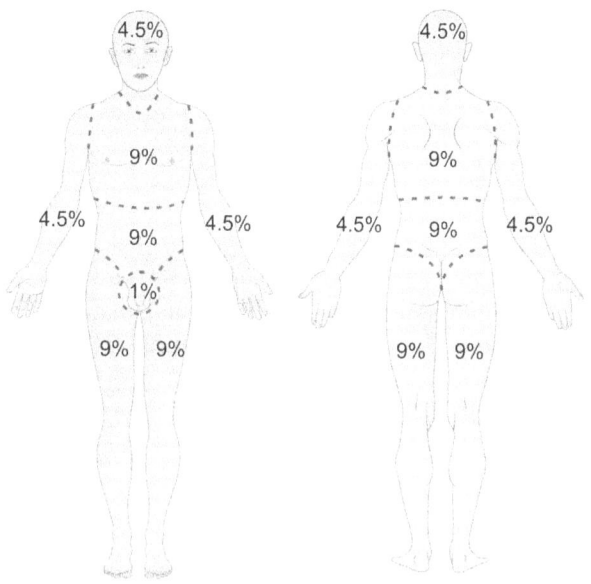

Fig. 9.2: Rule of nines.

treatment. Any burn larger than 2-3 cm (1 inch) diameter requires medical attention. The rule of nines is as follows:
- **Head:** 9%
- **Upper chest:** 9%
- **Upper back:** 9%
- **Arm:** 9% + 9%
- **Abdomen:** 9%
- **Lower back:** 9%
- **Legs:** 9% + 9%
- **Groin:** 1%

General Guidelines for Treatment of Burns and Scalds
- Avoid handling the affected area more than is necessary. See that hands are as clean as possible by washing them.
- Cool the burn area with cold water (15-25°C [59-77°F]) as soon as possible and continue till pain resolves.
- Do not use ice. Ice water can be used for cooling burns, but not more than 10 minutes.
- Avoid using topical creams, lotions or oil as they seal heat and can cause more damage.
- Do not remove burned clothing, leave blisters intact and do not break them.
- Cover the area (including burned clothing) with a prepared dry sterile dressing if possible, otherwise clean lint, freshly laundered linen or some similar material may be used.
- Bandage firmly except when blisters are present or suspected in which case bandage lightly.
- Immobilize the affected area by suitable means.
- Treat for shock.
- To treat skin or eye exposure to acid or alkali, first aid providers must immediately irrigate the skin, or eye with copious amounts of tap water. Apply a soft pad of cotton wool over his/her eye and keep the pad in position by using adhesive tape or bandage applied lightly.
- All electrical burns should have a medical evaluation.

First Aid Measures
- **Person's clothes catch fire**
  - Approach him/her holding a rug, blanket, coat, or table cover in front of oneself for protection, wrap it round him/her **(Fig. 9.3A)**, lay him/her flat and so smoothen the flames.

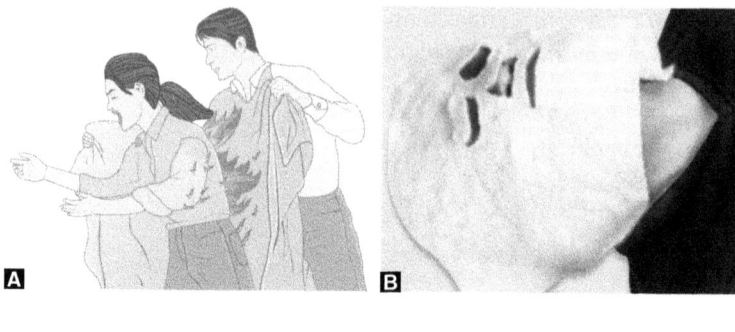

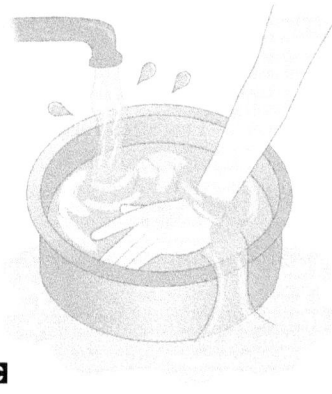

Figs. 9.3A to C: First aid for different types of burns: (A) Using a blanket to stop the burns; (B) Dressing shape in mask form; (C) Flooding acid burn area with water.

- In a major case, transport the patient to hospital as quickly as possible.
- The casualty will probably require an anesthetic so that ordinarily nothing should be given by the mouth.
- If medical aid is delayed for at least 4 hours, give water to drink which salt has been added in the proportion of half a teaspoon to two glasses (400 cc), with the addition of approximately half a teaspoon of bicarbonate of soda (if available).
- In a minor case, give large quantities of warm fluids. Preferably weak tea sweetened with sugar.

❖ **Face burnt**
  - Cut from a piece of clean lint, a dressing in the shape of a mask **(Fig. 9.3B)**, with a hole for breathing.
  - Maintain in position by a bandage as for fractured jaw.

- **Acid burnt**
  - Thoroughly flood the part with water.
  - Bathe the part freely with an alkaline solution, such as two teaspoons of baking soda (bicarbonate of soda) or washing soda (carbonate of soda) in one pint of warm water.
  - Apply the general rules for the treatment of burns, but remove contaminated clothing as quickly as possible to prevent further injury. Take reasonable precautions against burning oneself with contaminated clothing.
- **Alkali burnt**
  - If the burn is caused by quicklime, brush off any alkali that remains on the part.
  - Thoroughly flood the part with water.
  - Bathe the part freely with a weak acid solution, such as vinegar or lemon juice, diluted with an equal quantity of warm water.

Dry Burns and Scalds

Burns and scalds must be cooled as soon as possible in order to prevent further damage to underlying tissues and to alleviate pain, swelling and the possibility of shock. The most effective method of cooling is to flood the area gently with cold water.

Any clothing, which has been soaked in boiling fluid should be removed as soon as it begins to cool. Cooled, dry, burnt clothing should not be removed because doing so may introduce an infection:
- Very small burns or scalds can generally be treated on site.
- Friction burns, e.g., rope burns, should be treated as minor burns unless the skin is broken. If the skin is broken treat as for minor external bleeding.

General Symptoms and Signs
- Severe pain in and around the injured area.
- Redness and possible swelling of the area. Sometimes peeling of the skin and blisters, which may be broken.
- In deeper burns the skin may appear gray, pale or waxy or may be charred. There may be areas of numbness.
- Symptoms and signs of shock, which may be delayed. The degree of shock will relate directly to the extent of the injury.

First Aid Measures

Aims

- Reduce the effect of the heat.
- Prevent infection.
- Relieve pain.
- Minimize shock.
- Arrange immediate transportation to hospital, if burns are severe or extensive.

General Treatment

Minor burns and scalds:

1. Reassure the casualty: Place the injured part under slowly running cold water or immerse it in cold water for at least 10 minutes, longer if the pain persists or if no water is available use any cold harmless liquid such as milk or beer.
2. Gently remove any rings, watches, belts, shoes or other constricting clothing from the injured area before it starts to swell.
3. Dress the area with clean, preferably sterile dressings.
4. If in doubt about the severity of the injury—seek medical aid.

> **Note:**
> - Do not break blisters, remove any loose skin or otherwise interfere with the injured area.
> - Do not apply lotions, ointments or fat to the injury.
> - Do not use adhesive dressings.

For severe burn and scalds:

1. Lay the casualty down, protect the burnt area from contact with the ground, if possible. If the burnt area is still hot, carefully pour jugs of cold water or suitable cold liquid over the burnt area and continue until the pain has stopped.
2. Gently remove any rings, watches, belts or constricting clothing from the injured area before it starts to swell.
3. Carefully remove any clothing soaked in boiling fluid after it has begun to cool.

> **Note:**
> Do not remove anything that is sticking to a burn.

4. Cover the injured area with a sterile dressing or similar non-fluffy material, e.g., a freshly laundered sheet or pillow slip. A clean preferably new plastic bag may be used for an injured hand or foot. Secure with a bandage.

Note:
- Do not break blisters, remove any loose skin or otherwise interfere with the injured area.
- Do not apply lotions, ointments or fat to the injury.

5. For facial burns indoors, cool with water until pain is relieved; no cover is usually required. Alternatively make a mask from a clean, dry, preferably sterile piece of material (a pillow case is useful) with holes for the nose, mouth and eyes.
6. Immobilize badly burned limbs as for fractures.
7. To minimize shock, treat as for shock.
8. If the casualty becomes unconscious, open his/her airway and check breathing. Complete the C-A-B of resuscitation and place him/her in the recovery position.
9. Arrange immediate transportation to hospital maintaining the treatment position. Transport as stretcher case, if necessary.

Burns in the Mouth and Throat

Burns to the mouth and throat usually result from drinking very hot liquid, swallowing corrosive chemicals or inhaling very hot air. These injuries are very serious, because the tissues in the throat swell quickly and can close the airway making it difficult, if not impossible for the casualty to breathe. As a result, there is a real danger of asphyxia. In this situation it is particularly important to prevent the casualty panicking, these by worsening the situation.

Symptoms and Signs
- Casualty complains of severe pain in the injured area.
- Damaged skin around the mouth.
- Difficulty in breathing.
- Possible unconsciousness.
- Symptoms and signs of shock.

First Aid Measures
- Reassure the casualty.
- If he/she is conscious, give sips of cold water at frequent intervals.

- Remove any constricting clothing or jewelry from his/her neck and chest.
- If he/she becomes unconscious:
  - Open airway.
  - Check breathing.
  - Complete the C-A-B of resuscitation, if necessary.
  - Place in the recovery position.
- To minimize shock, treat as for shock.
- Arrange immediate transportation to hospital, maintaining the treatment position. Transport as a stretcher case, if necessary.

Chemical Burns in the Skin

Certain substances are irritating to the skin and contact with them can cause severe damage to the tissues. Eyes are particularly vulnerable. Apart from the local effects, a few chemicals may be absorbed through the skin and cause widespread and sometimes fatal damage within the body.

Strong corrosives and chemicals will be found in industry, but some household goods such as caustic soda, bleaches, household cleaners and paint strippers can cause chemical burns. While prompt action with this type of burn is important, one should always consider own safety before approaching the casualty.

Symptoms and Signs

- Casualty may complaint that skin is stinging.
- Skin may appear strained or reddened, blistering and peeling may develop.

First Aid Measures

Aims

- Identify and remove the harmful chemical as quickly as possible.
- Do not waste time looking for antidote, unless it is immediately available.
- Arrange immediate transportation to hospital.

Treatment

1. Flood the affected area with slowly running cold water for at least 10 minutes to prevent further damage to the burned tissues.
2. Make sure the water drains away freely and safely as it will be contaminated by the chemical, which caused the burn.

CHAPTER 9: Burns and Scalds

3. Gently remove any contaminated clothing while flooding the injured area; make sure one does not contaminate oneself.
4. Continue treatment for severe burns.
5. Arrange immediate transportation to hospital. Transport as a stretcher case if necessary.

Chemical Burns in the Eye

Corrosive chemicals, both liquid and solid can easily enter the eye and rapidly damage its surface, causing severe scarring and even blindness.

Symptoms and Signs
- Intense pain in the affected eye
- Damaged eye cannot tolerate light
- Affected eye may be tightly closed
- The eye may be reddened, swollen or watering excessively.

First Aid Measures
Aim: Wash away the chemicals as quickly as possible and arrange immediate transportation to hospital.
- Hold the affected side of the casualty's face under gently running cold water so that the water drains away from his/her face and not into his/her good eye.
  - If this is not possible, sit or lay the casualty down with his/her head tilted back and turn towards the affected side.
  - Protect the uninjured eye, gently open the eyelid of the affected eye and pour sterile water from an eye irrigator or a glass of tap water over it.

> **Note:**
> Both surfaces of the eyelids must be well irrigated for at least 10 minutes. If the eye is shut in a spasm of pain, pull the lids firmly, but gently open.

- Lightly dress the eye with a sterile eye pad or if this is not available, a pad of clean, non-fluffy material.
- Arrange immediate transportation to hospital.

Electrical Burns

A burn may occur when electricity of a sufficiently high current and voltage passes through the body. Much of the damage occurs at or close to the points of entry and exit but, while only small burns may be visible, damage to the underlying tissues may be considerable. Electric shock can also affect both breathing and heart action. The most dangerous causes of electrical burns are high voltage industrial machinery and lightning. Electricity in high voltage industrial cables can rump or 'arc' up to 18 m (20 d) and kill. So, do not approach the casualty unless, officially informed that the current has been switched off.

Severe injury may be caused by the passage through the body of an electric current. This may be due to contact with a line and naked wire, cable or rail or from a stroke of lightning. The immediate effect is shock, which may be relatively mild or so severe as to cause death (electrocution) depending on the strength of the current and on the path it takes in passing to arch through the body. Another result is burning and the burns may be severe and deep, especially with higher voltages. Electric injuries may occur:

1. In houses and offices, firm domestic apparatus with voltages up to 450 (alternating current).
2. In factories from equipment with voltages as high as 1,100 (alternating current).
3. Contact with a live-rail voltage in the region of 1,000 (direct current).
4. From overhead lines with high voltages of well over 100,000 (alternating current).
5. From lightning where the strength of current is immeasurable and the voltage may be many millions, e.g., standing under trees, in contact with metal railings or golf clubs.

Alternating currents are more dangerous than direct currents as the muscles are thrown into spasm causing the casualty to remain fixed in contact with the current. Moisture is a powerful conductor of electricity and when present, will facilitate the passage of the current. If the skin at the point of contact of earth is wet even the lower voltages may be dangerous. More important than the actual strength of the current is the path it takes through the body in finding its way to earth. Thus, a very strong current passing to earth through the lower limb might be less dangerous than a much weaker current crossing the chest as unfortunately it is likely to do, if it enters through the hand and arm. In these cases, there may be immediate fatal paralysis of the heart or more commonly a sudden stoppage of breathing from paralysis of the muscles of respiration. If the nerves controlling the heart and circulation escape, the heart may continue to function even though the breathing has stopped. It is for this reason that in electrical injuries the face is blue (asphyxia) rather than white and that artificial respiration may have to be carried on for a very long time. As long as the heart beats life may be saved.

Symptoms and Signs

- Redness, swelling, scorching or charring of the skin at both the entry and the exit points
- Possible unconsciousness
- Breathing and heart beat may have stopped
- Symptoms and signs of shock.

First Aid Measures

Aim: Separate the casualty from the source of injury, treat the burns and arrange transportation to hospital.

Treatment

1. Place a sterile dressing or pad of clean, non-fluffy material over the burn, secure with a bandage.

   Note
   Do not break blisters, remove any loose skin; do not apply lotions, ointments or fat to the injury.

2. To minimize shock, treat as for shock.
3. If the casualty becomes unconscious, open his/her airway and check breathing. Complete the CAB of resuscitation, if necessary and place his/her in the recovery position.
4. Arrange immediate transportation to hospital maintaining the treatment position. Transport as a stretcher case, if necessary.

   Electric injury is an emergency calling for prompt and intelligent action:

- Prompt action, if the casualty's life is to be saved.
- Intelligent action, if two casualties instead of one are to be avoided.

1. **Switch off the current:** If the switch cannot be found immediately and the supply is through a flexible cable the current may be cut off by removing the plug or even breaking the cable or wrenching it free **(Fig. 9.4)**. Do not attempt to cut the cable with a knife or scissor. It is impossible to switch off or break the current.

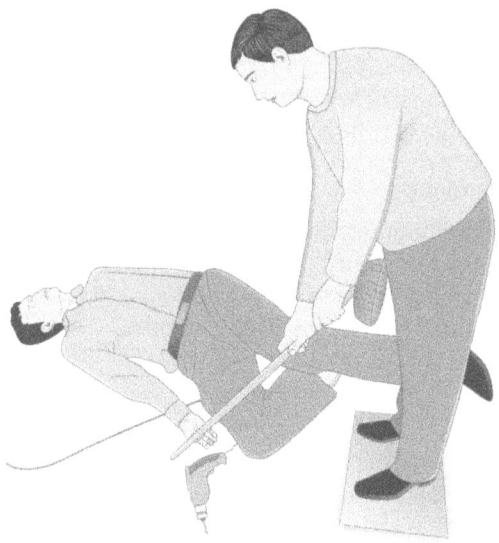

Fig. 9.4: Removing the electrical wire using a stick.

2. **Remove the casualty from contact with the current:** The greatest care is necessary; insulating materials must be used and they must be dry. With ordinary domestic apparatus rubber gloves are good and a dry cap, coat or other garment or a folded newspaper give fair protection. If possible, the rescuer should stand on some insulating material such as rubber-soled shoes or boots or piles of new papers.

With very high voltage, e.g., overhead lines, danger may exist even if the casualty is not actually in contact because the current may jump the gap (arcing). In these cases, the rescue should, if possible, be left to a properly trained electrical man although there is no danger, if the current is switched off. If expert help is not available, approach with great caution and keep as far away from any part of the electrical equipment as possible. Drag the casualty away with some non-conducting implement such as a dry walking stick, a dry board or dry rope.
3. Unless the casualty is breathing normally give artificial respiration for some hours if necessary.
4. Treat for shock (*refer* Chapter 3.3, topic on 'Shock').
5. Treat any burns.
6. Transfer to hospital or seek medical aid.

7. Even after apparent recovery the casualty should be seen by a doctor to ensure that all is well as casualties suffering from electrical injuries are liable to rephrase even when the effects have seemed to be mild.

Snow Blindness, Welder's Flash and Radiation

When the eyes are exposed to glare produced by the reflection of the sun on snow or concrete for too long, the cornea of the eye can be injured. This painful condition can take as long as a week to subside. It can easily be prevented by wearing dark glasses. This condition can also result from the ultraviolet light produced by welding. Most protective helmets and goggles give complete protection, but careless use may expose the eyes to a flash from an adjacent torch.

Signs and Symptoms

Signs and symptoms normally appear sometime after exposure to glare, welding flash or radiation.
- Casualty complains of intense pain in the affected eyes; may feel gritty.
- Affected eyes will be red, watering and sensitive to light **(Fig. 9.5)**.

First Aid Measures

- Cover the eyes and seek medical aid, if injury is severe.
- Bathe the eyes with cold water.
- Lightly dress both eyes with eye pads or similar pads of clean, non-fluffy material.
- If in doubt about the severity of the injury, seek medical aid urgently.

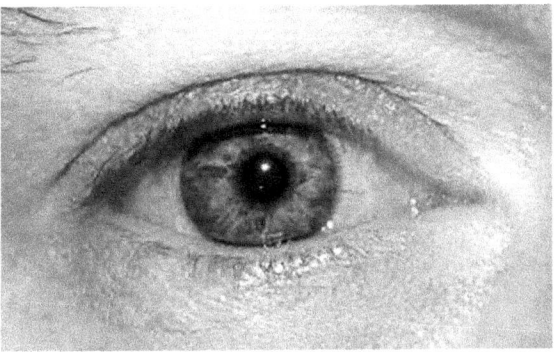

Fig. 9.5: Eyes affected by snow blindness.

REVIEW QUESTIONS

LONG ESSAYS

1. Define burns. Explain the different types of burns.
2. Describe electrical burns in details.
3. First aid management of dry burns and scalds.

SHORT ESSAYS

1. Chemical burns in the eye.
2. First aid measures for acid and alkali burns.
3. General guidelines for treatment of burns and scalds.
4. Explain snow blindness including first aid measures.
5. Management of burns in mouth and throat.

Poisoning, Bites and Stings

CHAPTER 10

10.1: POISONING

CHAPTER OUTLINE

- Definition of Poison
- Mode of Poison Entry into the Body
- Poison Action and Effects
- Poison Determination by First Aider
- General Rules for Treatment of Poisoning
- Household Poisons
- Drug Poisoning
- Alcohol Poisoning
- Industrial Poisoning
- Carbon Monoxide Poisoning
- Food Poisoning
- Swallowed Poisons
- Agriculture Poison
- Common Poison in India

INTRODUCTION

Poisoning is a life-threatening condition that is caused by exposure to harmful substances intentionally or unintentionally. Exposure can occurs at home or at workplace, it is therefore important to understand the types and nature of the poison including their antidote, protective equipment and emergency first aid management. The most common types would be ingestion and inhalation.

DEFINITION OF POISON

A poison is any substances that, if taken into the body in sufficient quantity, can cause temporary or permanent damage. It is also defined as any substance, which when taken into the body in sufficient quantity is capable of injuring health or destroying life. It may be taken either accidentally or intentionally.

MODE OF POISON ENTRY INTO THE BODY (FIG. 10.1.1)

1. **Inhalation**: Through the nose into the lungs by inhaling household or industrial gases, chemical vapors or fumes from fires, stoves,

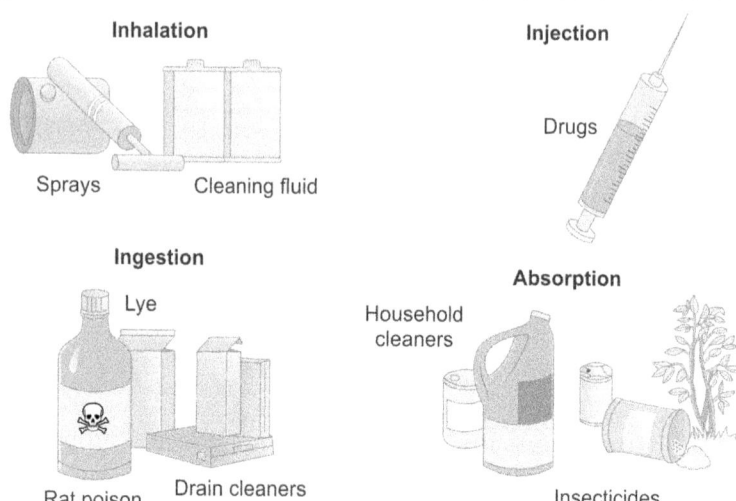

Fig. 10.1.1: Poison mode of entry with examples.

faulty appliances and petrol engine exhausts. This is put first because gas poisoning causes more deaths then all other poisons combined

2. **Ingestion:** Through the mouth by drinking or eating poisonous substance.
3. **Injection:** By injection into the skin as the result of bites from some animals, insects, poisonous fish or reptiles, or by hypodermic syringe.
4. **Absorption:** By absorption through the skin through contact with poisonous sprays such as pesticides and insecticides.

POISON ACTION AND EFFECTS

1. When poison enters into the body poisons acts in various ways. Once entering to the blood-stream, some poisons work on the central nervous system (CNS) preventing breathing, heart action and other vital processes. Other poisons act by displacing the oxygen in the blood and preventing its distribution to the tissues.
2. Swallowed (ingested) poisons also react directly on the food passages, resulting in vomiting, pain and often diarrhea. Corrosive poisons may severely burn the lips, mouth, gullet and stomach, thus causing intense pain.

3. Gas poisoning occurs mainly from breathing household gas or the fumes of fires, stoves, motor exhausts or the smoke generated from large fires or explosions. Life is endangered by asphyxia. The casualty may appear deceptively well unless severely poisoned when they will be unconscious with difficult breathing.
4. Swallowed poisons exert their dangerous effects by:
   a. Directly on the food passages causing retching, vomiting, pain and often diarrhea poisons in this class include metallic poisons, poisonous fungi and barriers, and contaminated decomposing food. Particularly severe symptoms are caused by the corrosives (strong acids, alkalis and disinfectants), which burn the lips, mouth, gullet and stomach, and cause intense pain.
   b. On the nervous system after absorption into the blood usually causing deep unconsciousness (coma) and sometimes asphyxia. The most important of these poisons are alcohol (spirits, wine and beer) taken in excessive amount, and the many drugs taken as tablets, or draughts to relieve pain (e.g., aspirin and preparations containing opium derivatives) or to produce sleep (e.g., the barbiturate drugs). All person's unconscious from poisoning by drugs are seriously ill; this also applied to individuals who are insensible from alcoholic intoxication (dead drunk). A few poisons act on the nervous system by causing delirium (e.g., belladonna) or fits (e.g., strychnine and prussic acid).
5. **Infected poisons:** These poisons are infected by hypodermic syringe, by bites from poisonous reptiles or rabid animals, or by stings from certain insects. As a result, life may be endangered through coma and asphyxia.

POISONING DETERMINATION BY FIRST AIDER

These vary depending on the nature of the poison and the method of entry into the body (*refer* **Table 10.1.1**).
- Information from the casualty or an onlooker suggesting contact with poison.
- Try to ascertain what was involved and if swallowed, when and how much was taken.
- The presence of a container near the casualty determine the types of poison consumed by the person.

Table 10.1.1: First aid treatment for corrosive poisons.

Poison	Common source	First aid treatment
Acids (strong)	• Dispensaries laboratories • Garages • Industries	• Do not make the casualty induce vomiting. • Give plenty of water to dilute the acid and if possible, 2 tablespoons of chalk, milk of magnesia, plaster or white-wash, to a pint of water
Alkalis (strong)	• Dispensaries laboratories • Some industries or in the home (ammonia)	• Do not make the casualty induce vomiting • Give plenty of water to dilute the alkali, add if possible 2 tablespoons of vinegar, orange, lemon or lime juice to a pint of water
Disinfectants, e.g., carbolic acid, Lysol, izal and cresol	• Hospitals • Dispensaries or in the home	• Do not make the casualty induce vomiting • Give 2 tablespoons of Epsom salts in a pint of water or in a tea cup full of medicinal paraffin
Other poisons		
Arsenic	In some weed killers, rat poisons and sheep dips	• Make the casualty induce vomiting • Give the soothing drinks
Aspirin		• Make the casualty induce vomiting • Give water to which add two teaspoons of bicarbonate of soda to the tumbler may be added • Give strong tea or coffee
Carbon monoxide from gas stoves or exhaust fumes		• Apply artificial respiration • Give oxygen, if available can be obtained in some garages and chemists
Medicine		
Chloral, Luminal sleep tablets, veronal and the other barbiturates		• Make the casualty to vomit • Give a dessert spoon of Epsom salts in a tumbler of water and give hot coffee • Keep the casualty awake
Metals		
Lead	In some paints and hair dyes	• Make the casualty induce vomiting • Give a dessert spoon of Epsom salt in a cup of water

Contd...

Contd...

Poison	Common source	First aid treatment
Mercury	• Corrosive • Sublimate • Calomel, some teething powders	Give white of egg in water followed by milk, then make the casualty vomiting
Opium and morphia	• Hospitals • Dispensaries	• Make the casualty induce vomiting • Give a few crystals of permanganate of potash dissolved in a tumbler of water • Give hot coffee • Keep the casualty awake
Paraffin petrol	• Houses • Garages • Industry	• Make the casualty induce vomiting • Give copious draughts of water
Phosphorus	Some rat poisons	• Make the casualty induce vomiting • Give water copiously with, if possible, a few crystals of permanganate of potash to each tumbler • Never give oils
Prussic acid	• Cyanides used in photography • Electroplating oil of bitter almonds	• Act at once, make the patient induce vomiting
Strychnine	Some vermin killers	• Make the casualty induce vomiting • Do not restrain movements, if breathing stops apply artificial respiration

❖ Casualty may be delirious and have convulsions (without previous history of such conditions).

GENERAL RULES FOR THE TREATMENT OF POISONING

1. Send for medical aid at once giving brief particulars including, if possible, the suspected cause. Preserve for examination:
   a. Any remaining poisons.
   b. Any box, carton, bottle or other container, which may help to identify the poison.
   c. Any vomited matter.

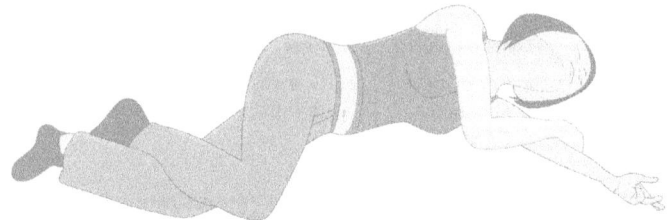

Fig. 10.1.2: Recovery position.

2. If the casualty is unconscious:
   a. Place him/her in the recovery position or prone position with the head turned to one side and not resting on a pillow. This will help to prevent vomited matter from entering the windpipe and keep the tongue clear of the airway. It also makes it easier to apply artificial respirations at once should this be necessary. If, however, there is much retching and vomiting the three-quarter prone position (recovery position **Fig. 10.1.2**) may be better, i.e., the casualty is on his/her side with the upper most leg bent at hip and knee or a pad supporting the chest.
   b. Start artificial respiration instantly, if the breathing is feeble or unduly slow. Keep it up till the doctor takes charge.
3. When poison has been swallowed and the casualty is conscious:
   a. Get rid of the poison by making him/her vomit. Trigger the gag reflex by inserting a spoon or two fingers into the throat, or if this method fails, give an emetic, i.e., two tablespoons of salt to a tumbler of water, preferably tepid. Do not induce vomiting:
      – When the casualty is unconscious.
      – When the lips and mouth are burned. Corrosive acids and alkalis cause yellow or grey stains on the skin, lips and mouth, which are easily recognizable.
   b. Neutralize the poison by giving an antidote. An antidote is a substance when reacts with the poison and makes it harmless. For example, when an acid has been swallowed an alkali such as chalk or milk of magnesia should be given.

   For some poisons there are special antidotes. In certain factories there may be particular hazards and, in these cases, special antidotes are usually kept readily available. Instructions for their administration should be prominently displayed.
   c. Dilute the poison by giving copious draughts of water. This will help to lessen the irritating effect and to delay absorption

in strong concentrations. It will also replace fluid host by vomiting.
   d. Give soothing drinks such as milk (at least one pint), barely, water, raw eggs or flour beaten up with water.
4. Special treatment to be given when the poison is known and shown. The quantities mentioned below to be reduced by a half for children between 2 and 8 years of age and reduced to a quarter for infants under 2 years. Where instructions are given to make the casualty vomit, it is assumed that he/she is conscious and is able to swallow. *Refer* **Table 10.1.1** for first aid treatment of corrosive poisons.

TYPES OF POISONS

Many substances found in and about the home can be poisonous. This includes liquid soap, some cosmetics, firelighters, white spirit, bleach, glue, rat poison, paint stripper, garden sprays and insecticides **(Fig. 10.1.3)**. Children are especially at risk from such materials, since

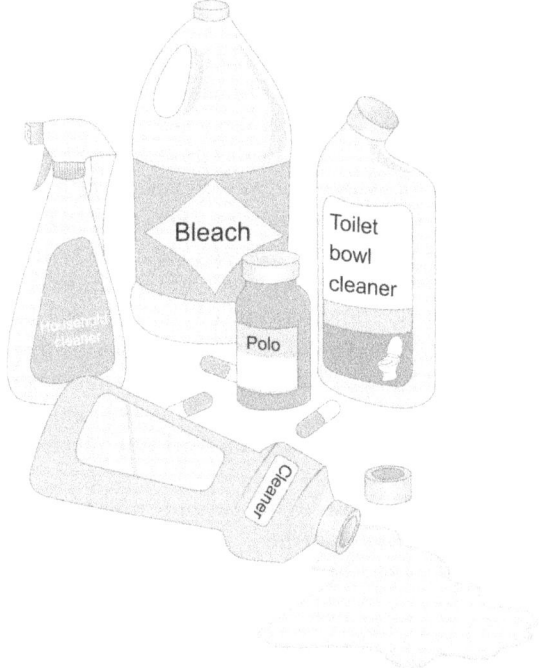

Fig. 10.1.3: Household poison.

they may not or cannot be aware of the consequences of eating or drinking them.

Risk of Poisoning at Home

- Poisonous substances in the home are medicines, household cleaning materials and garden insecticides can all be dangerous if eaten or drank, especially by children.
- Some of the more dangerous medicines include capsules and tablets, which looks as sweats, especially the colored ones, e.g., certain iron tablets tranquilizers and barbiturates.
- The symptoms and signs will vary according to the poison although vomiting and abdominal pain are likely to occur in most cases. Treat the casualty as for general treatment for poisons.

> **Note:**
> Always make sure that all bottles and jars containing poisonous substances are clearly marked and kept out of reach of children.

Poisonous Plants

Certain plants, around the gardens as well as in the wild are dangerous, if eaten and some may cause allergic reactions if touched. Children, in particular, are attracted by the bright berries of many of these plants and sometimes eat them. Laburnum *(Laburnum anagyroides)* **(Fig. 10.1.4A)**, deadly nightshade *(Atropa belladonna)* **(Fig. 10.1.4B)** and death cap fungus *(Amanita phalloides)* **(Fig. 10.1.4C)** are the more common examples of plants, which can poison the system.

The symptoms and signs of this type of poisoning are similar to those of food poisoning. The severity of the condition will depend upon how much of the plant has been taken. If it is suspected that a casualty has eaten a poisonous plant or berries, it is important that to maintain an open airway and transport the casualty to hospital immediately:

- Symptoms and signs of asphyxia and unconsciousness may develop.
- If the poison was swallowed, the casualty may begin retching or vomiting, or suffer from diarrhea.
- Burns around the casualty's mouth.

> **Note:**
> A casualty attempting suicide may dispose of any evidence, which would aid diagnosis.

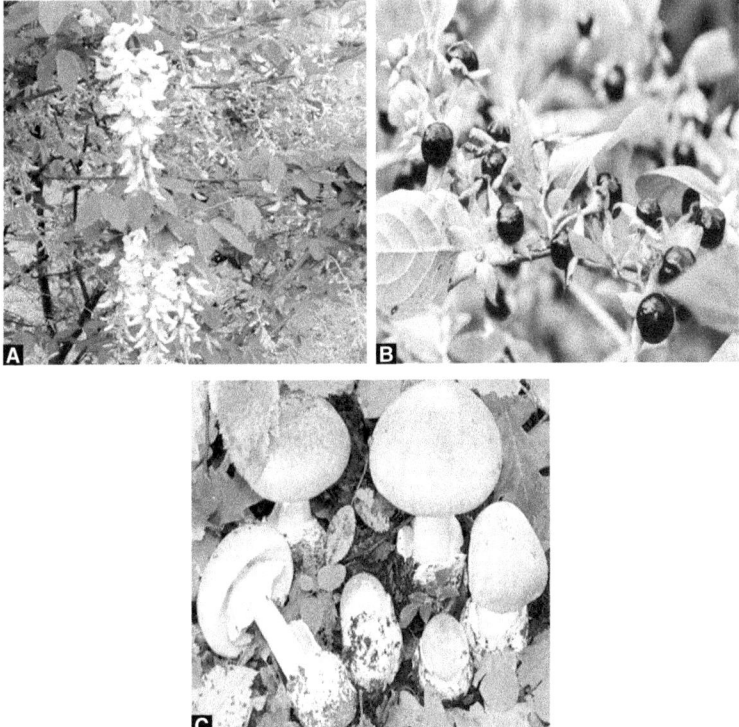

Figs. 10.1.4A to C: (A) *Laburnum anagyroides*; (B) *Atropa belladonna*; (C) *Amanita phalloides*.

First Aid Measures for Household Poisons

Aims: Maintain an open airway, breathing and circulation, and get the casualty to medical aid or hospital as soon as possible.

- Quickly ask the conscious casualty, what has happened. Remember that he/she may lose consciousness at any time.

> **Note:**
> Do not attempt to induce vomiting.

- If casualty lips or mouth show signs of burning, cool them by giving water or milk to sip slowly.
- Place casualty in recovery position even if he/she is not unconscious (he/she may vomit).

- If consciousness is lost, follow resuscitation immediately (*refer* Chapter 6.2).

> **Note:**
> Take care not to contaminate oneself with any poison that may be around the casualty's mouth.

- Arrange urgent transportation to hospital, send any samples of vomit and any containers such as bottles or pill boxes found nearby along with the casualty.

Drug Poisoning

Drug poisoning is a condition caused by an accidental drug overdose or drug abuse. Drug abuse may be broadly defined as the self-administration of a drug in a manner, i.e., not in accordance with approved medical or social patterns. Drug can be inhaled, swallowed or injected into the body. A regular drug abuser may show signs of continuous use of hypodermic injections. These marks will usually be on the front of the forearm near the elbow, although other places are also used. The veins in the area will become inflamed and infected.

Drugs commonly abused are narcotics (e.g., heroin) depressants (e.g., barbiturates and tranquilizers), stimulants (e.g., amphetamines) and hallucinogens [e.g., lysergic acid diethylamide (LSD)]. In addition, there is solvent inhalation (e.g., glue, sniffing).

Signs and Symptoms

Signs and symptoms will vary according to the drug and the quantity taken. Vomiting will not always appear immediately, but one should watch for it. The pupils of the eyes may be abnormally dilated or contracted.

Narcotics

Narcotics are usually injected, but can be taken in tablet form or inhaled:
- Breathing becomes difficult and eventually will cease.
- Casualty may have injection marks on the front of one or both arms.

Depressants

- Breathing will be shallow.
- Casualty's skin will feel cold and clammy.

- ❖ Pulse will be weak and rapid.
- ❖ Possible unconsciousness.

Stimulants

- ❖ Casualty will be excitable and sweating profusely.
- ❖ Casualty may be suffering from tremors and hallucinations (*see* objects and hearing sounds, etc.) not actually present.

Hallucinogens (Drugs Causing Hallucinations)

- ❖ Casualty will be anxious and sweating.
- ❖ Casualty may be behaving strangely and suffering from hallucination.

Aspirin Overdose

- ❖ Casualty has abdominal pain and may be vomiting; vomit may be blood stained.
- ❖ Casualty may be depressed and drowsy.
- ❖ Casualty may complain of ringing in the ears (tinnitus).
- ❖ Difficulty in breathing.
- ❖ Casualty will be sweating profusely.
- ❖ Pulse will be full.

Treatment

- ❖ Follow the general treatment for poisoning.
- ❖ Arrange urgent transportation to hospital and be prepared to resuscitate.

Alcohol Poisoning

Alcohol is a drug that depresses the CNS. It affects different people in different ways. One drink usually only produces a slight change in mood. As the intake continues, however, the drug affects the areas of higher reasoning within the brain those that control restraint and judgment. As the concentration of alcohol in the blood increases, the behavior of the drinker becomes exaggerated, and coordination will be impaired. Eventually, the mental and physical abilities are deeply disturbed and unconsciousness will develop.

Signs and Symptoms

- ❖ Casualty's breath may smell of alcohol.
- ❖ Casualty may be vomiting.

❖ Casualty may be partly conscious or already unconscious. If unconscious, rouse him/her, but will lapse into unconsciousness again quite quickly.

Early stage of unconsciousness	Later stage of unconsciousness
• Deep breathing • Moist and flushed face • Full and pounding pulse	• Rapid but weak pulse • Shallow breathing • Dry face and bloated look • Bloodshot eyes and dilated pupils

Note:
If there is a head injury, it may alter the symptoms and signs (*refer* Head Injury given in Chapter 4.2).

First Aid Measures

Aims: Ensure an open airway, arrange transportation to hospital, if the casualty is unconscious.

❖ Maintain an open airway (*refer* Chapter 6.2).
❖ If the casualty becomes unconscious or vomiting is likely, then place him/her in the recovery position.
❖ Complete the CAB of resuscitation, if necessary.
❖ If in doubt about his/her condition arrange transportation to hospital.

Industrial Poisons

Some people may be in contact with dangerous chemicals or gases at their workplaces as a result of the failure of a chemical plant, for instance, spillage of corrosive substances. Amongst the most common industrial poisons are the gases. These are usually classed as:

❖ Irritants (e.g., ammonia and nitrous fumes)
❖ Asphyxiants (e.g., carbon dioxide)
❖ Toxic gases (e.g., carbon monoxide and hydrogen cyanide gas)
❖ Toxic vapors (e.g., those given off by volatile chemicals such as carbon tetrachloride or trichloroethylene).

There are so many different poisonous substances in use that it is impossible to give a comprehensive list. Any factory using potentially dangerous chemicals or gases must display notices indicating any special action to be taken in case of accidents.

Safe Handling of Industrial Poisoning Guidelines for First Aider
- Contact responsible works official.
- Always obey any safety regulations to avoid further injury to both oneself and the casualty.
- Remember that any casualty suffering from the effects of gas or toxic fumes needs air.
- Take great care to prevent oneself being overcome by any fumes that remain in the area.
- Never attempt to rescue a casualty trapped in an enclosed space unless one is equipped with, and practiced in the use of breathing apparatus and life-lines.

Carbon Monoxide Poisoning

Carbon monoxide is a colorless, odorless gas. Its fumes are dangerous because carbon monoxide replaces the oxygen in the blood (it is more readily absorbed by the blood than oxygen). A casualty may require prolonged artificial ventilation to clear completely. The most common sources of carbon monoxide are fumes from partially burnt fuels and motor engine exhausts. Danger arises if an exhaust system is defective or if an engine is left running in an enclosed space. Enter a gas-filled room to rescue a casualty only if you are not in any danger and if you can get out again easily. Make sure you have backup help. A rescue rope around the waist is a useful precaution.

Signs and Symptoms
- Similar to general signs and symptoms of asphyxia.
- Headache.
- Color may be normal but will deeper to cherry pink as the level of carbon monoxide in the blood rises.
- Confused and uncooperative.
- Breathing is difficult or may have stopped.
- Unconsciousness may develop.

> **MANAGEMENT**
> **AIM:** Restore fresh air and adequate breathing. Arrange transportation to hospital.
> - Open any doors and drag the casualty to safety, if possible.
> - If the casualty is unconscious, open his/her airway and check breathing.

- Perform CPR and place the patient in recovery position.
- Check breathing rate, pulse and level of responsiveness at 10 minutes interval.
- Arrange transportation to hospital.

Note:
- Carbon monoxide is produced by incomplete combustion of any fuel and carbon dioxide may be found in mines and similar enclosed spaces.
- Butane and propane are used at home and in industry for heating, lighting or refrigerating, and can leak from faulty connections.

Food Poisoning

Food poisoning is caused by food becoming contaminated by bacteria and being stored or cooked incorrectly. Food poisoning can occur when cooking utensils, which are made of brass or copper and are not properly tinned, are used for cooking. Copper is poisonous and is ingested with the food causing severe symptoms, viz. diarrhea, vomiting or abdominal cramps, within hours of eating the poisoned food. Poisoning may also occur with the same signs and symptoms, when poisonous fruit or other vegetables are eaten or poisonous drugs are taken.

The most common bacteria are staphylococci, which multiply in the food and produce a poisonous substance (toxin) or *Salmonella*, which multiply in the bowel and cause dysentery like illness. *Salmonella* is infectious and can be passed through poor personal and kitchen hygiene.

Signs and Symptoms (Fig. 10.1.5)

Signs and symptoms depend upon the type of poisoning.

Staphylococcal Poisoning

These symptoms and sign will appear within 2-6 hours of eating contaminated food, the symptoms such as:
- Nausea and vomiting
- Abdominal pain and headache.
- Diarrhea may develop at a later stage.
- Symptoms and signs of shock.

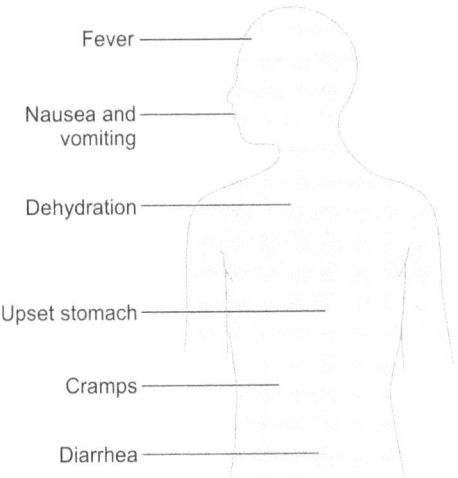

Fig. 10.1.5: Common symptoms of food poisoning.

Salmonella Poisoning

The signs and symptoms of *Salmonella* poisoning may appear within a few hours of eating or be delayed for a day or two:
- Fever
- Diarrhea
- Nausea and vomiting.
- Abdominal pain.
- Signs and symptoms of shock.

Main causes of diarrhea are:
- Food, which has been contaminated by flies or dirty food handlers.
- Polluted water supply, which has been in contact with human or animal excrement.
- The consumption of rotten or bad foodstuff.
- The utilization of badly tinned cooking utensils.

First Aid Measures

- *Aim*: Seek medical aid.
- Follow the general treatment for poisoning.
- Make sure the casualty rests.
- Give plenty of fluids to drink.
- If in doubt, arrange transportation to hospital.

Swallowed Poisons

The poison may be swallowed accidentally (e.g., children eating berries or pills; unlabeled or wrongly labeled bottles, or it may be an attempted suicide).

General Rules for Treatment of Swallowed Poisoning

- Get medical aid as soon as possible.
- Keep carefully any bottle, glass, etc. which might have contained the poison and any vomit.
- Unless there is a stain around the mouth, make the patient vomit.
- If the patient is conscious, give fluids to dilute the poison, and the antidote, if known (an antidote is a substance, which neutralizes the poison, making it harmless).
- Give soothing drinks, e.g., milk, white of egg, rice water.
- Treat for shock, keep the patient warm and loosen tight clothing.
- If unconscious, put the patient in semi-prone position.
- Watch the breathing and if necessary, give artificial respiration.

Type of Swallowed Poisons

Irritants

Irritants are substances, which irritate and inflame the tissues. For example, certain food items, fungi, berries, kerosene oil, arsenic, lead and mercury.

First Aid treatment

- Make the patient vomit by triggering the gag reflex or by giving the emetics, e.g., strong salt water (a tablespoon to a glass or 200 mL of water).
- Give plenty of fluids, e.g., rice water, milk or plain water. This will dilute the poison and make up for fluids lost through vomiting and diarrhea.

Corrosive Poisons

Corrosive poisons are strong acids, strong alkalis and disinfectants. These poisons burn the lips, mouth, esophagus and stomach. They cause severe pain and shock. The burned tissues may swell and cause breathing difficulty and there may be blood-stained vomit.

CHAPTER 10: Poisoning, Bites and Stings | 203

First Aid Treatment

- Do not induce vomiting; it might result in perforation of the stomach wall.
- Give two glasses of milk or water.
- Give an antidote if known:
  - If acid has been swallowed, give an alkali such as sodium bicarbonate or white-wash, two tablespoons to a pint of water.
  - If alkali such as ammonia has been swallowed, give a weak acid such as lime juice or vinegar, two tablespoons to a pint of water.
  - If a disinfectant has been swallowed, give magnesium sulfates two tablespoons in a pint of water or a cupful of liquid paraffin.
- Give soothing drinks, e.g., milk, white of egg, rice water or oil.
- Treat for shock.
- If the throat is swollen, give only cool fluids and apply hot fomentations to the neck.

Nerve Poisons

Nerve poisons affect the nervous system. Examples of these are:
- Morphia, opium, chloral, luminal, etc. which cause unconsciousness.
- Belladonna, atropine, alcohol, which cause restlessness delirium, rapid pulse and respiration, and later unconsciousness.
- Strychnine cyanide, which causes severe spasms of the muscles with arching of the back.

First Aid Treatment

- Make the patient vomit, immediately before the drug is absorbed.
- Give strong black coffee or tea, unless there are spasms.
- If an antidote is known, give it, e.g., for morphia give potassium permanganate solution.
- If there are spasms or delirium, keep the patient quiet in a dark room.
- In the case of poisons, e.g., morphia, artificial respiration may be needed.

Agricultural Poisons

Certain weed killers and insecticides used in agriculture as sprays for crops can give rise to dangerous poisoning through careless handling

or accidental contamination. Two kinds of poisoning occur, one of which closely resembles heat stroke. In the second kind, asphyxia may develop rapidly. Warning symptoms are giddiness, nausea, blurred visions and tightness of the chest. Signs may include:
- Slow pulse.
- Contracted pupils.
- Sweating.
- Bluish discoloration of the face and lips.
- Unconsciousness.
- Possible convulsions.

Treatment

Artificial respiration, which may have to be repeated or continued for a long time. As the doctor may wish to give a special antidote by injection, the first aider should give the suspected causes of the condition when sending for medical aid.

Common Poisons in India

Arsenic and opium account for the largest number of deaths from poisoning in India. Arsenical poisoning is the more common of the two, except in Bengal, which is an opium-eating country. Arsenic is the chief homicidal poison, while opium is the favorite of suicides.

Arsenic Poisoning

Common white arsenic in the crude form appears as lumps resembling white earthen ware and is easily obtainable in bazaars all over India. It is imported from the Persian Gulf and is used for preserving skins and woodwork, for destroying vermin and as a medicine. It is powdered down and being practically tasteless it is easily mixed with sweets and food. Being fatal in small doses, it is the most common homicidal poison.

Symptoms

- Are those of a violent irritant in which there is always an interval of ½–1 hour after taking arsenic.
- Burning pain in the stomach with vomiting and purging of blood-stained matter followed by numbness and cramps in the muscles. After large doses, collapse and shock precede death from coma.

Treatment
* General rules for treatment of poisons. Give an emetic white of egg or warm ghee to drink.
* In severe cases, give treatment for shock, i.e., hot bottles and stimulants.

Datura Poisoning
Datura poisoning is the third most common poison in India coming, however, a long way after arsenic and opium in frequency. The crushed seeds of *Datura* or thorn apple are administered in food and drink by criminals, with intent to rot rather than to kill.

Symptoms
* Those of belladonna poisoning, coming on fairly rapidly after partaking.
* Dryness of the throat, flushing of the face with a hot dry skin, and widely dilated and fixed pupils are typical.
* Difficulty in swallowing occurs with restlessness.
* Purposeless movements with muttering delirium lead on to conditions of coma, with death from failure of heart and respiration. The pupils remain widely dilated throughout and for days after recovery, which may take place.

Treatment
* General rules for poisoning, give an emetic, prevent hypnosis by flicking with towels or cold douching.
* Stimulate by hot coffee or a tablespoonful of brandy.
* Apply warmth and artificial respiration, if necessary.

Indian Hemp Poisoning
Indian hemp is available in the form of:
1. *Bhang*, which is the powdered leaves and small stalks.
2. *Ganja*, the dried flowering tops, which are smoked in a pipe.
3. *Charas*, which is the resinous juice, expressed from leaves and branches.

It is not a common cause of death and is used as an individual vice and as an intoxicant preparatory to robbery. The effects are those of a brain stimulant followed by narcosis. In the stage of stimulation, mental excitement is produced with hallucinations said to be pleasant. Laughing, singing and wild delirium are common results, while in some cases, there are violent homicidal tendencies, in which addicts run amok. Drug is sometimes taken by assassins to induce courage, or administered to them for the same purpose.

Symptoms
The pupils are dilated, the pulse full and slow, and there is general tingling of the skin. Giddiness gives place to stupor, coma and death.

Treatment
The treatment is same as of *Datura* poisoning.

Aconite Poisoning
Aconite is a most virulent poison, but fortunately not commonly employed in India. It is readily obtainable in Indian bazaars and sold as the dried shriveled root of the plant. It is used by native Hakims (or medicine men) for certain fevers and it is sometimes added to some of the country spirits as an extra intoxicant. Primitive hill tribes use aconite as dressing for their poisoned arrows.

When poisoning by aconite is met with, it is usually accidental, but homicidal poisoning is not unknown. The crushed root is mixed with tea, or cooked with food in these cases. The effect is first to stimulate sensory and motor nerves, with paralyzing effect later, in which the centers for the heart and respiration become involved. The mind remains unaffected.

Symptoms
- Tingling of the lips, tongue and throat with marked salivation appear first.
- Numbness in the limbs and whole body, followed by loss of power.
- The pulse and respiration become feeble and irregular leading on to a state of collapse.

Treatment
- Give an emetic and keep the patient in recovery position.
- Counteract collapse with stimulants strong coffee by mouth.
- Hot bottles and warmth in severe cases.
- Massage of the limbs relieves numbness.
- Artificial respiration may be required.

SOURCES OF VARIOUS POISONS, CLINICAL FEATURES AND FIRST AID MEASURES

Refer **Table 10.1.2.**

CHAPTER 10: Poisoning, Bites and Stings

Table 10.1.2: Sources of various poisons, clinical features and first aid measures.

Poison	Source	Clinical features	First aid
Strong acid	• Factories • Automobile • Repairing garages • Cotton mills • Dispensaries	• White stains, burning in throat abdominal pain, irregular respiration, weak pulse lowered body temperature, vomiting hematemesis	• No induction of vomiting • Olive oil, ghee, paraffin oil, barley water, milk of magnesia, white of an egg
Strong alkali	• Factories • Dispensaries	As with strong acid poisoning	No induction of vomiting lemon juice, vinegar, milk, egg yolk and olive oil.
Carbon monoxide	• Garages • Monoxide closed rooms with cool burning inside	Headache, cherry red flush, mental confusion, fever, convulsions, coma	Remove to a place with fresh air, artificial ventilation if necessary.
Iodine	• Medicine cupboard • Dispensaries • Industry	• Burning in mouth and abdomen • Excessive salivation nausea, vomiting, diarrhea	Starchy foods.
Kerosene	Household	Smell of kerosene nausea, vomiting convulsions and coma	Avoid aspirations into windpipe during vomiting.
Potassium permanganate	• Medicine cupboard • Dispensaries • Industry	• Brownish discolor 'Bates' mouth breathlessness, jaundice • Breathlessness Jaundice, oliguria	Activated charcoal.
Aspirin	• Dispensaries • Chemist's shop • Household	• Burning, pain in abdomen and vomiting • Hematemesis	Baking powder induce vomiting

Contd...

Contd...

Poison	Source	Clinical features	First aid
Mercury	Dispensaries	• White stains in mouth floor, pain in throat, difficulty in talking and breathing • Diarrhea	Egg white, arrow root
Morphine	Illicit drug trade	• Dizziness respiratory depression cyanosis • Hypothermia pinpoint pupils • Low blood pressure • Coma	Curd, butter milk, lemon juice
Strychnine	Ayurvedic doctors	• Dizziness, • Disorientation • Coma	Curd, butter milk, lemon juice, milk of magnesia
Sedatives	• Chemist shop • Household medicine • Cupboard	• Sleepiness • Disorientation • Coma	• Milk of magnesia, tea, coffee • If conscious, keep awake

REVIEW QUESTIONS

LONG ESSAYS

1. Mention mode of entry of poison into the body. Explain the action and side effects of poison.
2. Explain household poisoning.
3. Describe food poisoning with its management.

SHORT ESSAYS

1. General rules for treatment of poisoning.
2. Drug poisoning and its first aid measures.
3. Agriculture poisoning.
4. Arsenic poisoning and carbon monoxide poisoning.
5. List various metal poisoning and their first aid measures.

10.2: BITES AND STINGS

Chapter Outline

- Insects
- Spiders
- Snakes
- Scorpion Sting
- Bee, Wasp and Hornet Stings
- Jelly Fish Sting
- Portuguese Man of War
- Sea Urchin Sting
- Cone-Shaped Shells
- Coral Cuts
- Snow Blindness, Welder's Flash and Radiation
- Rabies and Anti Rabies Treatment in India

INTRODUCTION

Not all bites or stings are the same. Most of the bites and stings can be treated at home but a person bitten by an insect, spider or a snake, have to take different steps to apply the right first aid and seek proper medical assistance. It is also found that some bites and stings can transmit disease causing bacteria, viruses or parasites.

INSECTS

Nearly everyone has had an insect bite or sting at one time. Most bites or sting, whether from mosquitoes, flies, bees or wasps, results in a mild reaction to the venom or other protein that the insect injects into one. This can result in redness, minor swelling, pain and itching at the site of the bite or sting. Some people develop a severe allergic reaction to an insect sting, often from a bee or wasp.

Severe Reaction of Insect Bite

- Abdominal cramps
- Nausea and vomiting
- Swelling of the face, lips or throat
- Hives
- Breathing problems
- Shock.

FIRST AID MANAGEMENT OF INSECT BITE

- If the stinger is still in the skin, remove it by gently scraping across the skin with a flat-edged object, e.g., a credit card.
- Use **RICE** method of treatment. R- Rest, I- Ice, C- compression, E- Elevation.
- Wash the area with soap and water.
- Place a cold compress or an ice pack (wrapped in a cloth to protect the skin) on the sting or bite for about 10 minutes to reduce pain and swelling.
- Apply calamine lotion, an antihistamine cream, or a paste of baking soda and water to the area several times a day until itching and pain are resolved.
- Raise or elevate the affected area to reduce swelling.
- If there are signs of a severe allergic reaction, then ask someone to call for medical helps or emergency number if you are alone.
- Ask the person whether he/she carries an epinephrine injector, and if so, assist him/her to use it according to label directions.
- Help the person to remain calm and lie quietly with the legs elevated. If vomiting occurs, turn the person onto his/her side to prevent choking. Do not give them anything to drink.
- If the person becomes unconscious and stops breathing, begin cardiopulmonary resuscitation (CPR), and continue until medical help arrives.

Note:
- A severe, whole body allergic reaction is called anaphylaxis.
- If one has ever had a severe reaction to an insect sting, should request a medication called epinephrine from your doctor.
- Epinephrine acts quickly on the body to raise the blood pressure, stimulate heart, and improve swelling and breathing.

SPIDERS

Most spider bites are harmless, but symptoms can be noticed several hours or a day after the bite. The symptoms of spider bite is similar to an insect bite, such as redness, swelling, pain or itching. However, two kinds of spiders that can cause a more serious reaction are the black widow and the brown recluse.

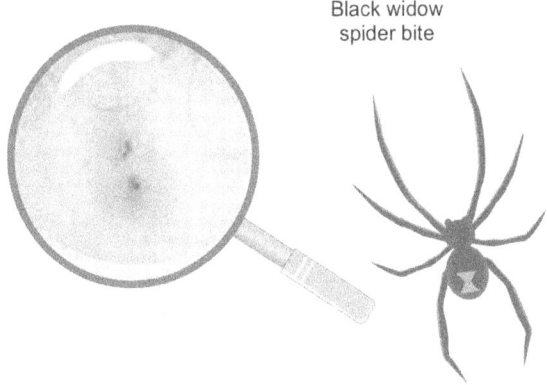

Fig. 10.2.1: Black widow spider.

Black Widow Spider

The black widow spider is about a half-inch long. It has a black body with a red hourglass marking on the underside of its abdomen (**Fig. 10.2.1**). Some black widows have red spots on the upper surface of the abdomen with crosswise red bars on the underside. Black widow spider venom causes problems with the nervous system.

Symptoms can be seen within few hours and it includes:
- Intense pain at the site of the bite.
- Chills or fever.
- Abdominal pain.
- Nausea and vomiting may be noticed.

Brown Recluse Spider

The brown recluse spider is larger than the black widow spider about an inch in length. It varies in color from a yellowish tan to a dark brown (**Fig. 10.2.2**). It has a violin shape on the surface of the upper body, with the base of the violin toward the head and the neck of the violin pointing toward the rear.

The brown recluse spider bite causes damage to the skin at the bite's area. About 8 hours following the bite, symptoms appear which includes:
- Redness.
- Intense pain.

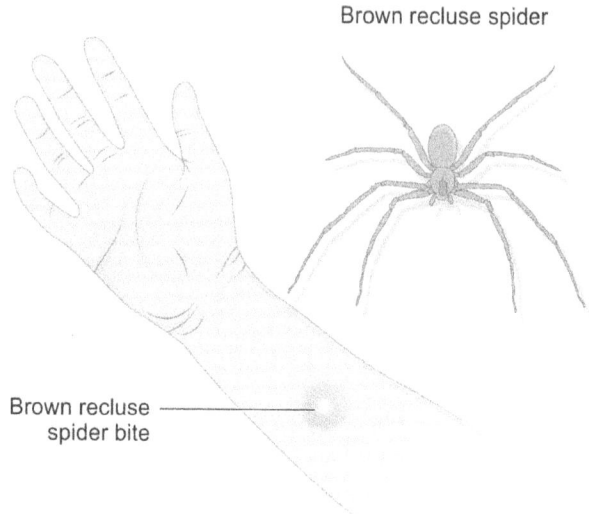

Fig. 10.2.2: Brown recluse spider.

- Development of a blister.
- When the blister breaks down, a deep ulcer is left in the skin.
- Fever, rash and/or nausea as well as the potential for an infection in the ulcerated skin area.

General First Aid Measures for Spider Bite

- First aid care is similar to that of an insect bite.
- Wash the area with soap and water.
- Apply tourniquet above the bite so that poison is limited to body parts.
- Place a cold compress or an ice pack (wrapped in a cloth to protect the skin) on the sting or bite for about 10–15 minutes to reduce pain and swelling.
- Elevate the bite area. Do not attempt to remove the venom.
- Apply calamine lotion, an antihistamine cream, or a paste of baking soda and water to the area several times a day until itching and pain are resolved.

FIRST AID CARE FOR A BROWN RECLUSE OR BLACK WIDOW SPIDER BITE
- Clean the skin with soap and water.
- Help the person remain calm to reduce the spread of venom; do not apply a tourniquet.
- Apply a cold compress or ice pack wrapped in a cloth to protect the skin.
- Get the victim to medical care as soon as possible. If possible, catch the spider or take a picture to help medical personnel identify it.
- Bite area should be clean daily with povidone-iodine solution and soaked 3 times a day in sterile salt water (saline).
- Hospitalization is required for people younger than 16 years and older than 60 years.

SNAKES

Snake bites are punctured wounds caused by the fangs of snakes. As far as the treatment of the wound is concerned, it is dealt with as a minor wound. However, in India, there are several poisonous snakes and unless you see the snake and are able to identify whether or not it is poisonous, you should always assume that the snake is poisonous. *Refer* **Tables 10.2.1 and 10.2.2** for types of poisonous snakes in India.

Table 10.2.1: Poisonous vipers land snakes found in India.

Russell's viper (Daboia)	• Found all over India • Longest and most poisonous viper • Varies from 1 to 5 feet in length • Reddish brown in color • Three parallel chain along back and sides • Body is of diamond-shaped blotches edged with white
Echis carinatus (Phoorsa)	• Found within Northern India • Seldom exceeds 2 feet in length and is less dangerous than 'Russell's viper • Dark white blotches on the top of its arrow-shaped head, outlined in black
Pit viper (Ancistrodon)	• Tree viper found in Ceylon and the hilly districts of Southern India • Named on account of the pit between eye and nostril • It may be 3 feet in length, is not very formidable • Seldom causes death

Table 10.2.2: Poisonous Colubrines land snakes found in India (See **Fig. 10.2.3**).

Common cobra (naga)	• Found all over India and the Himalayas • Long, cylindrical bodies up to 6 feet in length • Hooded and with spectacle markings on the hood
King cobra (hamadryad)	• Found in lower Bengal, Assam and Burma • May be 15 feet in length • Most poisonous of all Indian snakes
Krait (Bungarus)	• Found in Northern India and Sind • Two types: Common krait and banded krait • Common krait may measure 4 feet in length and has a series of white arches over the back, well-marked towards the tail • The banded krait sometimes measures 6 feet and yellow in color with black rings or bands encircling the body

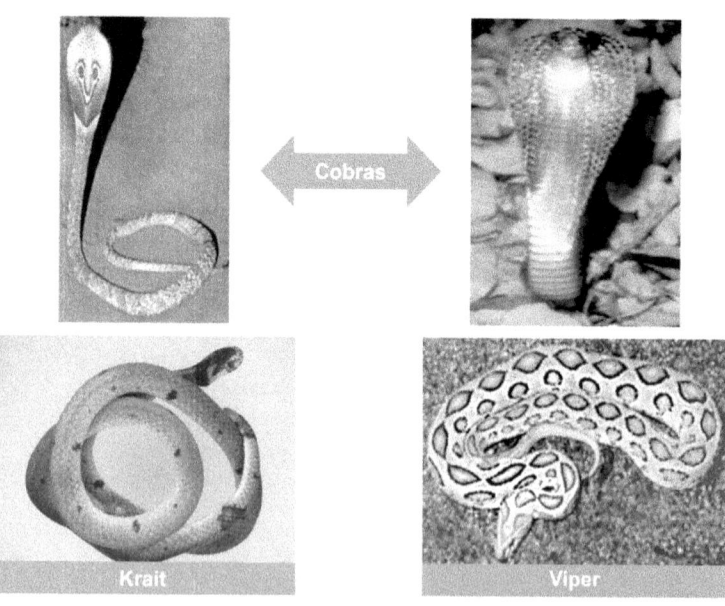

Fig. 10.2.3: Poisonous snakes commonly found in India.

Effects of Snake Venom

Viper	Colubrines
• It rapidly acts on blood and blood vessels • Local reaction of marked discoloration and hemorrhage round the punctures • Vomiting and collapse • Dilated pupils • Local sloughing and gangrene round the bite after recovery • Paralysis is rare	• Rapidly absorbed nerve poison • Severe pain follows the bite, with nausea and vomiting • Onset of paralysis of the legs is rapid • Poison ascends rapidly to the brain with paralysis of the face muscles and dripping from the mouth • Pupils are contracted • Respiration is rapidly extinguished

Signs

- Patient will tell you that he/she has been bitten by a snake
- Punctured wounds produced by the snake's fangs are clearly visible
- Patient may show signs of poisoning, e.g., bleeding or paralysis
- Signs of shock.

Symptoms

- Disturbed vision.
- Nauseated or already be vomiting.
- One or two small puncture wounds with sharp pain and local swelling.
- Breathing may become difficult or fail altogether.
- Salvation and sweating may appear in advanced stages of venom reaction.

Symptoms of a poisonous snakebite vary depending upon the snake, but can include:

- Weakness
- Dizziness
- Fainting
- Convulsions
- Nausea
- Vomiting
- Diarrhea
- Loss of muscle coordination
- Rapid pulse
- Swelling in the area of the bite

❖ A poisonous snakebite is a medical emergency. Quick treatment can minimize symptoms and aid in recovery.

Treatment

If snakebite complication occurs:
1. Give salt water, i.e., add five to six teaspoon salt in 200 mL of water and mix well.
2. Make the victims to drink, repeat this treatment hourly for 6 hours.
3. After 6 hours repeat the treatment once in 4 hourly for six times. This will nullify the snake venom complications.

First Aid Measures

Aims

❖ Reassure the casualty
❖ Prevent absorption of venom
❖ Arrange urgent transportation to hospital.

First Aid Measures for Snakebite

1. Summon medical help immediately.
2. Call for emergency services (112 for India).
3. Help the person to remain calm and lie quietly.
4. Movement can spread the venom more rapidly, so try to keep the body still, especially in the bitten area.
5. Tie a piece of cloth (at least within 1 hour) or a tourniquet, tightly above the bite to prevent the venous blood return, i.e., it should be tight enough to prevent the blood flow through the veins, but not tight enough to prevent the blood flow in the arteries **(Fig. 10.2.4)**.
6. Remove constricting jewelry or clothing around the bitten area, as swelling may occur.
7. Loosen the tourniquet for 1 minute in every 20 minutes.
8. Keep the bitten limb hanging down. Do not raise the bitten area above the level of the heart.
9. If there are symptoms of shock, such as dizziness, weakness, pale and clammy skin, shortness of breath and increased heart rate, have the person lie quietly with his/her feet elevated about 12 inches.
10. Cover him/her with a blanket to maintain body warmth.

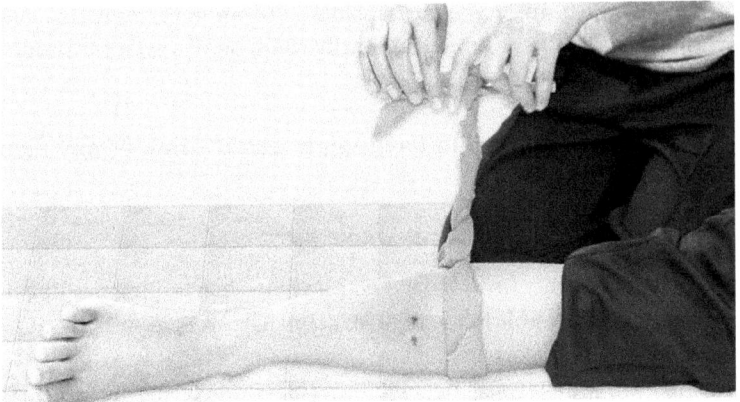

Fig. 10.2.4: Tying piece of cloth above the snake bite.

11. Examine the wound. If there are no fang marks the snake was not poisonous. If there are fang marks, try to get the patient to hospital immediately, an antivenom injection given in time may save his/her life.
12. If there is doubt and cannot get the patient to hospital quickly:
    a. Wash the wound with lukewarm water, with potassium permanganate added, if available.
    b. Sterilize a knife or blade in a flame and make a cut 1 cm deep in the form of a cross over the bite.
    c. Suck out the liquid (poison), using a piece of plastic over your mouth to protect yourself or suck out of the wound and spit it out. If the bite is on the arm, the patient can suck his/her own wound.
    d. Apply potassium permanganate crystals on the cut.
    e. Apply a clean dressing.
    f. Treat for shock.
    g. Refer to the nearest government hospital.
    h. If breathing fails, do artificial respiration.

Note
If by any chance the poison is swallowed, it does not do any harm.

Steps Not to Take
- Do not endanger yourself by trying to capture the snake.
- Do not cut or suck the area of the snakebite.

- Do not wash the snake bite (residual venom at the bite area can help medical personnel to identify the type of snake for proper treatment).
- Do not apply cold to the bite.
- Do not give the victim anything to eat or drink or any pain medication.

Examination of Snakes and Snake Bites

The first aid worker must have the knowledge of a trained naturalist. He/she should be able to distinguish at once between non-poisonous and poisonous snakes. Inspection of local site of bite can also help to identify snake's species. Local swelling, bleeding, blistering, necrosis suggests cobra bite. Minimum local changes indicate krait bite. Local bleeding suggests Nilgiri Russel's viper. Pain in abdomen and hyper peristalsis indicates krait bite.

Examination of the snakes must be done systematically as follows:
1. Examination of belly, top of the head, side of the face and lastly, the back.
2. Scales—large or small, are continuous with those of back and sides, and uniform across the belly.
3. Combination of small scales and transverse shields are seen on belly surface, but the transverse shields do not monopolize belly surface.
4. Transverse shields extend completely across from side-to-side occupying entire belly surface to the tail.
5. Top of head is arrow shaped. Broader than rest of the body, which it joins by a constricted neck. Head covered with small scales, common to all vipers, except pit viper.
6. Top of head is oval, smaller than rest of the body and streamlined without demarcation of neck covered with a big shield. If neck passes into expanded hood, then it is cobra; common cobra has spectacles, king cobra without spectacles.
7. Examination of side or face.
8. Shield on side of face. Tip-tilted nose with well-marked 'pit' between eye and nostril is 'pit' viper.
9. Absence of 'pit', probably krait.
10. Central row of large shields occupy midline of back, with foregoing features, can be regarded as a krait.

SCORPION STING

In many parts of India scorpions are common and scorpion stings are likely to occur. The person got stung, usually a child who is unaware of the dangers of scorpion lurking in dark places, complains of severe pain at the site of the sting and shows signs of shock. The scorpion sting is poisonous and if the child is small or physically weak it may produce serious results. If severe the patient may have cramps, sweating and possibly convulsions.

Signs and Symptoms
- Pain followed by numbness and tingling sensation in the sting area.
- Abnormal head, eye, and neck movements.
- Signs of shock.
- Increased saliva production.
- Sweating.
- Restlessness.

First Aid Measures
- Examine the site of the sting.
- Look for signs of shock, particularly in small children.
- Wash the area with soap and water.
- Apply a cold compress to the site of the sting or sodium bicarbonate paste (cooking soda paste).
- Tie a piece of cloth or a tourniquet above the stung area.
- Give hot drink and keep the patient warm.

BEE, WASP AND HORNET STINGS

Bee, wasp and hornet stings occur frequent in rural areas, especially if their nests are disturbed. The insects have a sting, which is left at the site of puncture and has to be removed. If a person is prone to allergies, a bee, wasp or hornet sting may be a serious condition because of the shock produced.

Signs
The site of the sting looks red, swollen and painful.

First Aid Measures
1. Remove the sting with a pair of forceps.
2. Apply cold compresses to the site.

3. A paste with sodium bicarbonate (cooking soda) or washing soda can be applied or if available antihistamine ointment.
4. Treat for shock.

JELLYFISH STING

The effects of Jellyfish sting vary from minor local reactions to large wheals, severe pain and sometimes death.

First Aid Measures

The first aid measures are as follows:
- Apply paste of sodium bicarbonate in water.
- Seek medical aid urgently, if symptoms are severe.

PORTUGUESE MAN-OF-WAR

The effects vary from slight stinging to cramps, nausea and difficulty in breathing.

First Aid Measures

- Swab the area with methylated spirit to which a little vinegar has been added to acidify it.
- Do not rub or apply fresh water or sand.
- Remove any gelatinous strands present in the flesh using cloth or soft paper, once symptoms subside.
- Seek medical aid in severe cases.

SEA URCHIN STING

The spine of the sea urchin can break off into the skin causing local burning and numbness. The wounds heal slowly, and the rate of infection is high.

First Aid Measures

- Wear gloves, while handling the sting
- Remove the spine
- Cover the wound with dry dressing
- Get medical aid.

CONE-SHAPED SHELLS

A snail-like creature is found in such shells. It injects a very potent poison through a minute hollow barbed harpoon. It can be fetal and there is no antidote. Such a shell must not be handled.

First Aid Measures

- Watch the patient's pulse and respiration.
- Give external cardiac massage and artificial respiration when necessary.
- Get medical aid urgently.

CORAL CUTS

Coral is razor sharp. The cuts are large and deep and get infected readily. They heal slowly and tend to form ulcers.

First Aid Measures

- Clean with methylated spirit
- Remove all foreign material from the cuts
- Cover the wound with sterile dressing
- Arrange for medical aid.

RABIES AND ANTIRABIC TREATMENT IN INDIA

Rabies is an acute infective fetal disease of dogs, jackals, wolves, horses, monkeys and other animals transmitted to man by bites and scratches from these infected animals, or by licks on preexisting abraded surface, e.g., rag, nails, cuts, etc. (**Fig. 10.2.5**). The poison

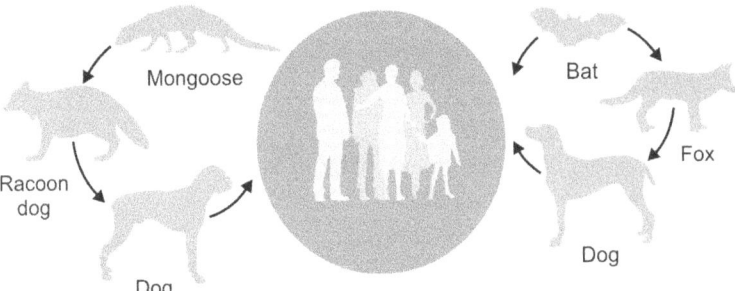

Fig. 10.2.5: Transmission of rabies.

or virus is probably an ultramicroscopic organism, contained in the saliva of these infected animals, which gains entrance to the system through the abraded skin surfaces of the victim.

Pasteur, about 1885, proved that rabies was essentially an infection of the central nervous system and that the pathway from skin to spinal cord was via terminal nerve endings and up along the parent nerve trunks.

Signs and Symptoms

In Human

Incubation period for Rabies is 15 days to 8 months. Symptoms appear in three stages:

1. **Invasion stage:** There may or may not be increased irritation or pain in the region bitten. Restlessness, insomnia, quickened pulse and slight fever are common.
2. **Excitement stage:** This follows in 1 or 2 days and lasts as long. Restlessness becomes intense with great mental excitement. Hypersensitiveness to any stimulus (e.g., noise, light, etc.) sets up distressing spasms of the muscles of the throat and respirations. Consciousness unfortunately remains clear.
3. **Paralytic stages:** This is the result of exhaustion, followed by heart failure in a matter of 1 or 2 days. The developed disease is incurable. In rapidly fatal cases, these stages may run into one another so closely as to be indistinguishable.

In Dog

A dog may be infective for 1 week before any symptoms develop. Two types in dogs are described:
1. Dumb rabies in which paralytic feature predominates.
2. Furious rabies in which irritation of the brain, with resulting excitement is most evident followed later by paralysis and of course death.

Symptoms is domestic dogs include:
- Stage of 'hot nose' and refusal of food, as an early sign.
- Restlessness ensues rapidly.
- Dog wanders about anxiously.
- Change of expression wrinkling of the eyebrows and a haunted look.
- Dog is apt to make unprovoked attack at this stage.

- Staggering gait, as a result of paralysis of the hind legs, appears early.
- General convulsions of all the muscles of the whole body precede deaths, occurs within 10 days.

Treatment

First Aid Measures—postexposure Prophylaxis

- Wash the whole abraded surface with the soap and water, detergent or povidone iodine for 15 minutes whether licked, scratched or lacerated.
- If pure carbolic acid (phenol) is available, paint carefully the abraded surface and edges of the wound by means of a match, or slip of split cane, dipped in pure carbolic acid. If the wound is penetrating do not omit to paint the sides of the depressions and probe to the bottom of each tooth mark. It stings on first application, but soon becomes anesthetic. Again, wash it with soap and water.
- Administer rabies immunoglobulin (RIG), if indicated.
- Vaccination—a course of potent and effective rabies vaccine that meets WHO standards.
- Collect all possible information regarding the circumstances of the bite.

Prevention

- Pre-exposure immunization for outdoor travelers and people living in remote areas with a high rabies exposure risk and limited local access to rabies biologics.
- Avoid keeping a domestic pet at home where there is young children. Children has the natural instinct to pet and fondle a pet dog and they court the disaster of dog bite.
- In districts where infected jackals roam about, it is not advisable to keep a dog at all.
- If the dog has a hot nose, is off color and refuses to eat food, in India, it should always be claimed up and the following precautions should be taken at this stage.
  - When giving the dog medicine, thick leather gloves to protect the hands should be used.
  - Chain the dog and release only when the dog's appetite and condition returns to normal.

- On the other hand, if suspicious symptoms develop, keep the dog chained up and away out of harm, and send for a doctor or veterinary officer.
- If there is a shadow of doubt they will order the dog to remain chained up for 10 days, especially if it had bitten anyone.
- No dog with developing rabies will survive 10 days (few will survive 5 days), so, even if the dog had bitten someone, and it is alive and well after 10 days it can be pronounced non-rabies to the relief of all concerned.

Note:
- Vaccinating dogs is the most cost-effective strategy for preventing rabies in people.
- Verify if the attack was unprovoked or merely the result of teasing the animal.
- If the bite is caused by a wild animal or stray dog, then it is best to assume that it was rabies.
- If the dog is known insist on the owner's chaining it up for the doctor's inspection.

REVIEW QUESTIONS

LONG ESSAYS

1. List the signs and symptoms of snake bite. Describe its first aid management in detail.
2. Define Rabies. Explain Antirabic treatment.
3. Signs and symptoms of dog bite in human. Explain its first aid management.

SHORT ESSAYS

1. First aid management of Insect bite.
2. Explain Frost bite.
3. First aid management of Scorpion sting.
4. Explain steps for identification of poisonous snakes.
5. Preventive measures for Rabies.

Frostbite and Effects of Heat

CHAPTER 11

CHAPTER OUTLINE

- Frostbite
- Effects of Heat
  - Heatstroke
  - Heat Exhaustion
  - Heat Cramps
  - Heat Rash
  - Sunburn

INTRODUCTION

Exposure to extreme hot or cold temperature can overburden the body temperature control system. Body heat is under the control of a temperature control center (thermostat) situated at the base of the brain, which automatically adjust the mechanism that keep the balance between loss and heat gain. Extreme heat or cold exposure can cause adverse health issues ranging from discomfort to death.

FROSTBITE

Frostbite is a condition in which local tissues are frozen, usually at the extremities. They become injured by prolonged constriction of the surface blood vessels as a result of exposure to extreme cold. As with heat burns, the damage may be either superficial or deep and the affected tissues may be destroyed. To prevent frostbite, wear adequate clothing and gloves, and leave as little skin exposed as possible.

Symptoms and Signs

- The affected areas (tip of nose, ears, fingers or toes) become pale at first, then waxy whites, later a mottled blue color and finally black **(Fig. 11.1)**.
- Blustering may occur.

Stages of frostbite

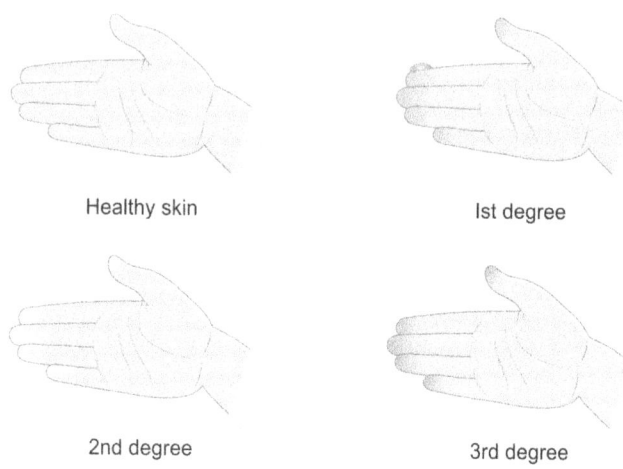

Fig. 11.1: Stages of frost bite.

- Casualty may complain of 'pins and needles' and intense pain, but the part gradually becomes numb and pain disappears as the freezing bites deeper.
- The skin feels hard and stiff.

Treatment

Aims

- Warm the affected area slowly and naturally to prevent further tissue destruction.
- Arrange transportation to hospital.

First Aid Measures

- Handle damaged area gently. Remove frozen covering carefully, together with rings or watches.
- Warm the part with own hands.
- If a finger is frost bitten, place the casualty's affected hand in his/her opposite armpit until normal color returns.
- Keep surroundings warm as soon as possible. If color does not return rapidly, warm gently by soaking the affected area in warm water (100-105° F) until it appears red and feels warm.

- As the part thaws out, the color will improve, and pain will return. Dry and dress the thawed area with dry gauze or wool and lightly bandage it.
- Elevate the limb to reduce swelling.
- Avoid breaking any blisters.
- Do not allow the affected area to refreeze.
- If authorized by a doctor, give the casualty two paracetamol tablets.
- Arrange transportation to hospital, transport as a stretcher case.

Note:
- Do not rub the area.
- Do not burst blisters.
- Do not heat the part with fires or hot-water bottles.
- Do not allow the casualty to smoke.

EFFECTS OF HEAT/ EXTREME TEMPERATURE

The effects of heat on the human body encompass a range of physiological responses and potential health outcomes. It is important to recognize the signs of heat-related issues, practice preventive measures, and respond appropriately to ensure personal safety and well-being in environments with elevated temperatures.

Effects of Heat

1. Heatstroke
2. Heat exhaustion
3. Heat cramps
4. Heat rash

Heatstroke

Heatstroke is the most serious condition that occurs due to extreme exposure to heat causing the body to overheat.

Signs and Symptoms (Fig. 11.2)
- High body temperature >103°F.
- Hot and dry skin.
- Rapid heart rate.
- Dizziness and headache.

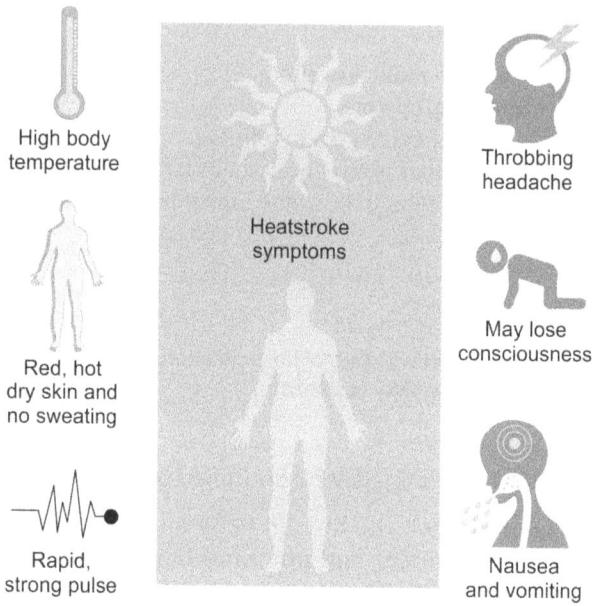

Fig. 11.2: Signs and symptoms of heatstroke.

- Nausea.
- Confusion.
- Loss of consciousness.

First Aid Measures
- Call emergency helpline number.
- Move/take the patient to a cooler place.
- Wrap the casualty in a cool wet cloth/sheet, keep pouring cold water over the sheets till temperature return to normal.
- Replace the wet sheet with dry sheet once temperature is normal.
- Do not give anything by mouth.
- Continuously monitor the casualty temperature and response level till help arrive.

Heat Exhaustion
When the body overheats from excessive heat exposure, particularly from physical activity in hot weather, heat exhaustion occurs.

Signs and Symptoms
- Sweating heavily.
- Cold, pale and clammy skin.
- Nausea and vomiting.
- Rapid and weak pulse.
- Tiredness and weakness.
- Muscle cramps.
- Dizziness and headache.
- Fainting.

First Aid Measures
- Move the casualty to cooler place.
- Loosen tight clothing.
- Pour water on the body till body cool down.
- Give him/her a sip of water.
- If the casualty starts vomiting, symptoms got worse and last for more than an hour call ambulance.

Heat Cramps
Heat cramps are excruciating, uncontrollable muscle spasms that typically happen during strenuous exercise in hot weather.

Signs and Symptoms
- Muscle spasm or pain commonly occurs in legs, arms or trunk.
- Heavy sweating during exercise.

First Aid Measures
- Move casualty to a cool place.
- Stop any physical activity or movement.
- Give him her water to drink.
- If the muscle spasm last longer than 1 hour, call ambulance or transport to nearby hospital.

Heat Rash
Heat rash is also called as Miliaria. Heat rash occurs when sweat is trapped/blocked in the sweat glands causing development of rash after a few days (**Fig. 11.3**).

Signs and Symptoms
- Red clusters or small blisters that look like pimples on the skin.
- Blisters are commonly found in neck, chest, groin and elbow.

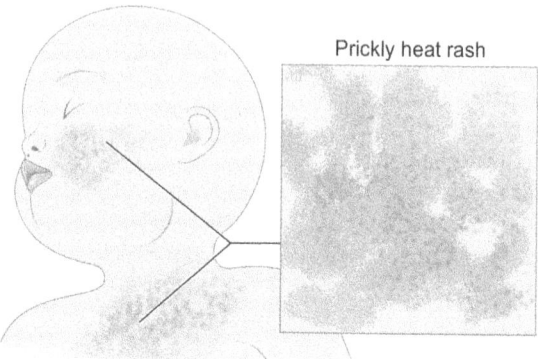

Fig. 11.3: Heat rash.

First Aid Measures
- Keep the skin dry.
- Avoid wearing synthetics cloths that cause irritation on the skin.
- Keep the rash dry by applying powder to the skin.
- If symptoms got worsen, contact dermatologist.

Sunburn

Direct exposure to the sun's rays may produce redness, itching and tenderness of the skin. It can vary from superficial burning to a more severe reaction in which the affected skin becomes lobster-red, blistered and painful. Over exposure to the suns' rays when it is very windy or the body is wet with sea-water or sweat can result in serious burns. However, sunburn can also occur even on a dull-overcast day in summer and in winter on high mountains, when skiing because of the ultraviolet light. Serious discomfort and even superficial burns with blister formation can be caused by the direct rays of the sun. In hot countries even short periods of exposure to the midday sun can cause quite severe burns. The first aider is unlikely to be required to treat sunburn as the symptoms and signs do not appear at once but may be delayed for some hours. Unless the condition is obviously trivial the casualty should be advised to see a doctor. If needed, the general rules for the treatment of burns and scalds should be applied.

Symptoms and Signs
- Skin will be red, tender and swollen with possible blistering.
- Affected skin will feel hot.

First Aid Measures

Aims
Remove the casualty to a cool place and seek medical help, if the burns are severe.

Treatment
1. Place the casualty in the shade. Cool his/her skin by sponging gently with cold water.
2. Treat for general effects of over-heating.
3. Give sips of cold water at frequent intervals.
4. For extensive blistering, seek medical aid immediately.

> **Note:**
> Do not break blisters.

REVIEW QUESTIONS

LONG ESSAYS
1. Describe frost bite and its first aid measures.
2. List the ill effects of heat and explain heatstroke in details.

SHORT ESSAYS
1. Heat exhaustion.
2. Heat cramps.
3. Heat rash.
4. Heatstroke.
5. Sunburn.

Community Emergencies 12

12.1: DISASTER MANAGEMENT

CHAPTER OUTLINE

- Definition
- Types of Disaster
- Causes of Disasters
- Effects of Disasters
- Management of Disasters
  - Phase of Disasters
  - Principles of Disaster Management
  - Phases of Disaster Management
  - Care of Disaster Victim: Triage, Victim Assessment, Mass Casualty Management, Coordinated Response of Emergency Services
- Disaster Management Agencies
  - National Agencies
  - International Agencies

INTRODUCTION

Disasters have existed ever since the existence of mankind. No community in the world is completely immune from both natural and man-made disaster. According to the Greek philosopher Empedocles, the universe consists of five elements—earth, fire, air, sun and water from which came the manifestation of violence such as earthquake, volcanoes, cyclone, droughts and floods.

Innumerable disasters strike the world every year resulting in many deaths and casualties. India is one of the most disaster-prone countries; the recent 'super cyclone' in Odisha has underlined the fact. The aftermath of the worst industrial disaster in the world 'Bhopal gas tragedy' on December 3, 1984, is still unfolding to this present day. The occurrence of Tsunami on December 2004 killed a total of 26,014 people. Disaster is very sudden and unpredictable; it can happen anywhere at any time and demands for 'immediate action' and gives no scope for planning. There is a need for adequate procedures to deal with disaster situations for every community of the world.

DEFINITIONS

Disaster is a natural or man catastrophe that cause helplessness and suffering, may involve physical injuries, loss of property and interruption of normal daily living:

1. Any occurrence that causes damage, ecological disruption, loss of human life and deterioration of health and health services on a scale sufficient to warrant an extraordinary response from outside the affected community.
 —World Health Organization
2. Disaster is catastrophe causing injury or illness simultaneous to at least 30 people who will require hospital emergency treatment.
 —Colin Grant, 1973
3. An emergency of such magnitude as to require extraordinary mobilization of the emergency services.
 —Rutherford, 1974
4. Any patient generating incident that results in overload of either existing personnel or existing supplies and equipment.
 —Holleran, 1992

TYPES OF DISASTERS

There are two categories of disaster according to their causes are natural and man-made (due to human error):

1. **Natural disaster:** They are due to violence of nature:
    a. Natural phenomena beneath earth's surface:
        - Earthquakes
        - Tsunamis
        - Volcanic eruption.
    b. Natural phenomena at earth's surface:
        - Landslide
        - Avalanches.
    c. Metrological/hydrological phenomena:
        - Windstorms—cyclone, typhoon and hurricane
        - Tornadoes
        - Hailstorms and snowstorms
        - Sea surges
        - Floods
        - Droughts.
    d. Biological phenomena:
        - Locust
        - Epidemics of disease.

2. **Man-made disaster:** They are due to human error:
   a. Caused by warfare:
      - Conventional warfare
      - Nuclear, biological and chemical warfare.
   b. Caused by accidents:
      - Vehicular: Plane crash and shipwreck, train and car accidents.
      - Collapse of building
      - Explosion
      - Fires
      - Biological
      - Chemical
      - Poisoning.

CAUSES OF DISASTER

I. **High wind flow phenomena:** High winds on storms are natural phenomena. These are characterized as follows:
   1. **Lightening:** Flashes of light in the sky are often seen during bad weather, when there is a collision of hot air masses with cold air masses. During lightening, squall—an unbroken line, about 40,000 feet long, develop in the sky and discharge nearly 30 million volts current per single flash of light within 1/10th of a second. These flashes of light seem to have the tendency to hit the higher places:
      a. It is safer to take refuge either inside a motor vehicle or in building wheel has a metal frame.
      b. Never stand under a tree during lightening.
      c. Remember the need for earthing in electrical circuit.
   2. **Hurricane:** These are tropical cyclones. These are low pressure winds formed over the ocean in areas where masses of warm and moist are formed. The wind blowing with velocity of 75 miles per hour (mph) is classified as hurricane:
      a. The greater number of hurricane occurs in the South Western Pacific Ocean. The Southern Indian Ocean and West Indies, etc.
      b. Many people living close to the sea are often caught in such disasters.
      c. Despite progress made in weather warning system, many lives and people continue to be lost every year. People who survive face the difficulties and stain of displacement.

d. Protective measures are important, e.g., shifting people to safer areas, educating people about boiling water for drinking and organizing mass immunization especially for the typhoid.
e. Such storms—high tides, heavy rains causing floods and create additional problem of shelter, food, drinking water, etc.

3. **Tornadoes:** These are moist, violent windstorms moving faster than hurricane in a 'funnel shape' and they build up a narrow path of destruction. Especially when it rises above and dips to the ground, it causes severe destruction where it hits. The extent of destruction depends upon the wind pressure, which many even exceed 300 km/h. Its destruction trail picks up animals, peoples, objects, automobiles and take them even a 100 miles away causing havoc to properties, injuries and death to people. In such disasters if injured are to be cared for at the scene, there will be problem of displacement.

4. **Blizzard:** These are severe blinding storm of fine snow blown by strong freezing winds. Many places in snowy regions are hit by such storms. These often cause transportation breakdown, communication breaks, and isolation of the affected people from others, loss of live stock and property. There will be difficulties in supplying food and other amenities to the area and also in shifting of casualties to the hospital, etc.

5. **Earthquakes:** It is a kind of faulty shifting of the earth layers leading to movement of its crust (fault) thus, causing tremors. Earthquake hit areas have number of problems such as arranging of food, clothing, lodging for survivors, control of epidemic, cleaning debris, linking communication and determining the soundness of the remaining structure, etc.

6. **Epidemics:** Weather differences often give rise to epidemics of various infections disease. A disease is said to be an epidemic when it is prevalent over larger areas at the same time, e.g., epidemic of cholera, typhoid, plague, influenza, polio, etc.:
a. Spread of many diseases is activated by poor personal hygiene, living under unsatisfactory sanitary conditions and contamination of drinking water.
b. In any outbreak of epidemic following are done to control the spread of further infection:
○ Quarantine.
○ Isolation of infection cases.
○ Enforcement of proper sanitary measures.

7. **Flood:** It is caused by high tide in coastal areas, brief torrential rains, constant rain extending over a longer period, deforestation of hills and mountains:
   a. People in these areas are faced with the dangers of losing lives and property; loss of shelters; displacement; lack of food and clothing; epidemics, etc.
   b. Flood control measures include:
      ○ Construction of hydro dams.
      ○ Planting of trees and vegetation to minimize erosion of soil.
8. **Transport accidents:** There is now high rate of automobiles accidents. Accidents of bus, trains involve larger number of people whereas in air crash, shipwreck, boat accident loss of life is usually more than the survival or injured. The management of such injuries depends upon the type of transport accident and number of people involved in an accident.
   Prevention
   – Proper maintenance of transport.
   – Use of road safely measures and protection devices minimize accidents and the severity of injury.
   – Educate people to develop the habit of observing and obeying rules and regulations laid down by the transport authorities.

II. **Fire:** Fire can be caused due to carelessness in handling fire objects such as throwing burning cigarettes or bidis, hot ashes, bursting of gas cylinders, electric sparks, spontaneous conflagration in forest or due to negligence of a man.
   Prevention
   * Practice safety measures, while using gas, electricity or for proper disposal of objects that can cause fire.
   * There are number of fire extinguishing devices now available, which can be installed in hotels, shops, offices and even houses. People concerned should know the use of these equipment.
   * Phone numbers '101' is dialed for calling fire force to extinguish in emergency.

III. **Explosion:** Explosions occurs in factories specially those engaged in manufacturing ammunitions, ships selling and storing crackers, mines, and oil wells. Example; explosive's bombs by militants and terrorists for destruction of planes, ships, buses, train, trucks, etc.

Prevention

- Making public aware of the hazards resulting from explosions.
- Enforcing the safety measures in factories, mines and those shops, which sell crackers, etc.
- Preventing the activities of antisocial elements.
- People are regularly educated through mass media to be observant and report any suspicious objects to the police.
- In certain fires connected festivals, e.g., Diwali, etc. The first aid team should be ready to meet any emergency.

EFFECTS OF DISASTER

Natural and man-made disasters present a serious threat to the health and welfare of all people throughout the world. Therefore, there is desperate need for community preparedness, particularly the healthcare system, especially hospitals, which should be prepared and equipped to mobilize all their facilities for maximum usage in whatever circumstances. Effects of disaster includes (**Fig. 12.1.1**):

- Loss of life.
- Physical injuries.
- Psychological trauma.
- Property damage.
- Environmental destruction.

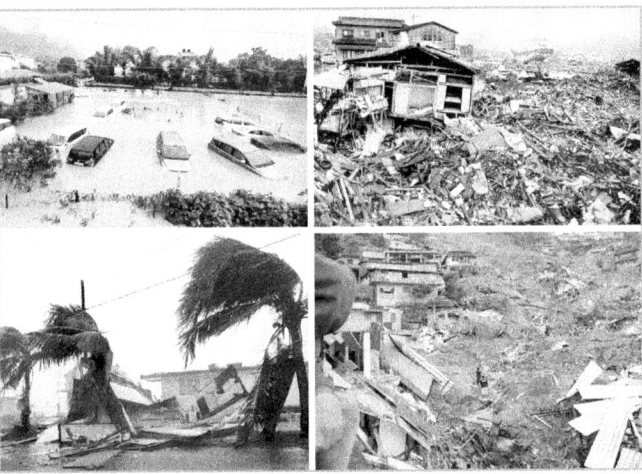

Fig. 12.1.1: Effects of various disasters.

MANAGEMENT DISASTER

AIM

To save as many lives as possible by providing the best possible medical care under those circumstances.

Phase of Disaster

The phases of disaster are the time periods of series of events, which vary according to the type of disaster. However, most include the:
1. Warning phase.
2. Threat phase.
3. Impact phase.
4. Inventory phase.
5. Rescue phase.
6. Remedy phase.
7. Recovery phase.

1. **Warning phase:** Some disaster give warning of their approach. In this, certain precautionary measures are undertaken to handle the disaster situation efficiently and effectively.
2. **Threat phase:** This is a critical decision-making period when one's activity is directed towards the survival action.
3. **Impact phase:** When disaster strikes, people may at first be stunned. Then they begin to realize the magnitude of the effects of disaster such as injury, death, destruction, etc.
4. **Inventory phase:** During this phase, one tries to find out what has actually happened to him/her. Victims may exhibit fear, anger, sorrow, depression, anxiety, apprehension and other emotions.
5. **Rescue phase:** During this post disaster period, the victim helps each other to cope and begin to help with the rescue, provide comfort to others and to re-establish shelter and other needs.
6. **Remedy phase:** The morale of survivors/victims usually picks up during this period as they work together with rescue personnel to get the community back on its feet. A spirit of cooperation often prevails. This phase is the longest post disaster period when reconstruction takes place.
7. **Restore phase:** In this phase, the individual regains the stability that they enjoyed prior to the disaster. The time required for a community to reach a state of equilibrium depends on the nature and intensity of disaster and the disaster relief available.

DISASTER MANAGEMENT

Principles of Disaster Management

The purpose of disaster management is basically to prevent and minimize death disability, suffering and loss. The following are the principles of disaster management:
1. Prevent the occurrence of disaster whenever possible.
2. Minimize the number of casualties, if the disaster cannot be prevented.
3. Prevent further casualties after the initial impact of disaster. The impact of many disasters is followed by unstable situations, which are dangerous to life and can be more dangerous than the original disaster.
4. Removal of victim to safety.
5. Provide first aid to the injured—prompt first aid must be initiated to prevent further damage/trauma and to prevent complications.
6. Evacuate the injured to the hospital/health center—the victims are to be transported carefully and as quickly as possible to the nearby hospital/health center to initiate medical management as soon as possible.
7. Provide definite medical care—efficient handling of a large number of casualties depends upon training of doctors and nurses, and the disaster preparedness of the concerned institution. However, health professionals should be trained to improvise. Where necessary with whatever available resources, so as to provide as effective and efficient care to the disaster victim as possible.
8. Promote reconstruction of the lives of victims—as soon as the medical and surgical procedures are over, rehabilitation of disaster victims must be undertaken through counseling services.

Disaster Management Phases (Fig. 12.1.2)

Disaster management phases consists of:
- Disaster preparedness
- Disaster response
- Disaster recovery
- Disaster mitigation

Disaster Preparedness

1. Preparedness is concerned with forecasting and working, education and training of population, organization for and management of

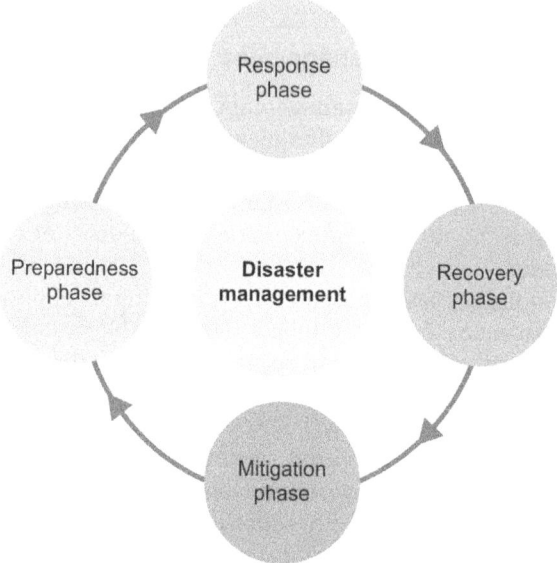

Fig. 12.1.2: Phases of disaster management.

disaster including preparation of operational plan, training of relief groups, ensuring adequate supplies and earmarking of necessary funds.
2. Preparedness is done through drills and exercise.
3. Preparedness must always be supported by the necessary legislation and indicates, which cannot be avoided.
4. Developing techniques for training, information transfer and hazard assessment.
5. Establish informal lines and ties between relevant groups.
6. Anticipating and communication about future dangers and hazards
7. Drawing up organizational disaster plans and integrating them in overall community disaster plan.

Disaster Response
1. Response starts immediately after the occurrence of disaster.
2. The duration of response and management of safety depends on the level of preparedness.
3. Response activities includes:
    - Implementing the plans conducted during disaster preparedness.
    - Conducting search and rescue mission.

- Focusing on the safety of the individual, family, community and including animals.
- Focus is also being laid on food safety.

Disaster Recovery

1. The recovery period focus on restoration of all damage/affected area to its previous functioning state.
2. Implementation of activities to reduce illness and excessive financial burden.
3. Reducing the risk of future disaster.

Disaster Mitigation

1. Actions taken during this stage include those aimed at reducing the catastrophes' causes, effects, and outcomes.
2. Some activities in this phase includes:
   - Securing house with ground anchors to prevent wind damage.
   - Installing vegetation to absorb water and creating water channels to redirect water.
   - Building levees or other long-term barriers to regulate flooding.
   - Investing on insurance policies.

Care of Disaster Victim

The goal of care in any situation is to provide the great chances of survival to the largest number of the disaster victims through a system of attending the most sick and serious injured victim first, then the ones who are less serious and could wait for some time to get medical attention. This system of prioritizing the victims is termed as 'triage'.

Disaster Triage

The goal of triage is to evaluate how serious the victim's condition is, set priorities, and choose the best course of action that will be beneficial to the person within the constraints of time and professional attention available at that location.

International Guidelines for Triage

- **Red**—Immediate care: Most urgent and high survival if attended immediately.
- **Yellow prime**—Beyond care: Regardless of urgency has poor survival rate.

- **Yellow**—urgent not immediate care: Can wait 45-60 minutes after stabilization.
- **Green**—minor care: Can wait until others have been attended.
- **Black:** Dead.

Triage priorities can change depending on the number of patients, types of injuries and number of emergency care providers at the spot. Patients do not always remain stable, and one has to update triage (*refer* **Table 12.1.1**). List of priorities in triage are given below:

Highest Priority

- Respiratory arrest, airway obstruction and severe breathing difficulties.
- Cardiac arrest.
- Uncontrolled severe bleeding.
- Severe head injuries.
- Open chest wounds.
- Open abdominal.
- Severe shock.
- Burns involving respiratory tract.
- Medical problems such as heart attack and poisoning.
- Unconsciousness.

Second Priority

- Severe burns
- Injuries to the spine
- Moderate bleeding
- Conscious patients with head injuries
- Multiple fractures.

Lowest Priority

- Minor bleeding.
- Minor fractures.
- Moderate minor burns.
- Obvious mortal wounds where survival is not expected.
- Obvious death.

Victim Assessment

Emergency medical care person should know about the vital status of the patient to diagnose the condition for an early treatment. One must be able to apply following information to the assessment and care of patients.

Table 12.1.1: Field triage flow chart using international convention color code—prime yellow green.

Color code	Red	Yellow prime	Yellow	Green	Black
Priority	Transfer immediately to a referral hospital with a medical escort in an equipped ambulance	Transfer only, after evacuating all red victims, with a medical escort in an equipped ambulance	Transfer to a referral hospital in ambulance with first aid escort	Transfer to an appropriate health care facilities by available vehicles without escort	Transfer to morgue
Urgency	Most urgent (fluids, intubation, Fasciotomy)	Urgent (constant, intensive care)	Urgent (IV line, drugs, immobilize fractures)	Not urgent (splint or dressing)	Non-urgent
Condition	Shock/hypoxia present/imminent	Deep shock, needs exceed available resources	Stable for 1 hour, can wait at field	Stable till end of response	No pulse or respiration No blood pressure or heart-beat
Injuries	Life-threatening	Catastrophic	Systemic effects, not yet life threatening	Localized	Fatal
Potential for survival	High after immediate care and transportation	Very poor	High after support treatment	Good	None
Examples	Intra-abdominal injury, shock status from any cause	Massive skull or chest injuries, extensive and severe burns	Heart attack, compound fractures, severe burns	Minor fractures, burns or wounds	Dead

Pulse

- Rapid and thready pulse is found in shock, loss, heat exhaustion, diabetic coma and falling of blood pressure.
- Rapid and full pulse is found in fear, overexertion, heat stroke, high blood pressure and early stages of internal bleeding.
- Slow and full pulse is found in stroke and skull fracture.
- Pulse is not found in cardiac arrest.

Respiration

- Rapid and shallow respiration is found in shock, heart problems, insulin shock and congestive cardiac failure.
- Deep and labored respiration is found in airway obstruction and chest injuries.
- Snoring is prominent in drug or alcohol abuse, partial airway obstruction.
- Coughing blood is common in chest wound, rib fracture and advanced tuberculosis (TB) lungs.

Blood Pressure

- High blood pressure is seen in chronic hypertension, head injury, severe pain, etc.
- Low blood pressure is noted in hypotension, shock, internal bleeding and chest injury.

Pupils

- Dilate pupils not responding to light is in cardiac arrest, unconsciousness, shock, bleeding, consumption of lysergic acid diethylamide (LSD) drug, etc.
- Constricted pupils are seen in morphine poisoning.

State of Consciousness

- Confusion is being noted in fright, anxiety, illness, head injury, drug abuse, alcoholism and epilepsy.
- Stupor is noted in severe head injury, stroke or drug abuse.
- Brief unconsciousness is seen in fainting, epilepsy and head injury.
- Coma is seen in stroke, anaphylactic shock, severe head injury, poisoning, diabetic coma, heat stroke, etc.

Paralysis

- One side of the paralyzed body is noted in stroke and head injury.

- Upper limb paralysis is seen in spinal injury of neck.
- Lower limb paralysis is noted in spinal injury along back.

Mass Casualty Management

- Do the best for the most promptly within the prevailing resources
- Triage
- Grade the care of casualties:
  - First aid
  - Lifesaving measures
  - Preparation for evacuation
  - Primary surgery.
- Limit the first aid activities at the disaster site for maintaining and restoring vital functions.
- Transport the victims.
- Work with confidence and coordination with other members of rescue team.

Tips for Disaster Rescuers

- **Be professional:** To stay to detect the victim's problems and needs.
- **Have a presence of mind:** Be prompt in any action, what normally a prudent person would do.
- **Talk with victims:** Acknowledge their individual existence, fears, questions and needs.
- **Listen to victims:** Reassurance often comes from having someone listening especially for victims who are panic, argumentative or overly active.
- **Provide needed care:** Both physical and emotional needs of the victim must be considered.
- **Provide food and drink:** Those who are allowed to take food and drink should be provided periodically. This will have a calming effect, provide assurance.
- **Design tasks for the victims:** Those who are injury free should be kept engaged by simple tasks, i.e., feeding, giving water to those who are helpless.
- **Keep victims together:** This will help the victims to think that he/she is not alone or a stranger during a disaster.

Coordinated Response of Emergency Services

Underservices coordination is the core of any disaster operation. Activities associated with disaster preparedness, mitigation and disaster response in a community has to be multidisciplinary in nature. Following are some of the emergency services, which should be coordinated at the onset of any disaster.

Police

The police department provides 24 hours service. Police are the first to get information about the onset of disaster and to reach to the site. They disseminate the information for the organization of an orderly rescue and relief operation. The task responsibilities of the police in disaster are:
- Control of traffic and crowd.
- Protection of life and property.
- Search and rescue operation **(Fig. 12.1.3)**.
- Warning and evacuation.

Firemen

Primary role of the firemen is to extinguish and prevention of fire **(Fig. 12.1.4)**. The tasks basically performed by the firemen are:
- Extinguishing and preventing fire.
- Rescue.
- First aid.

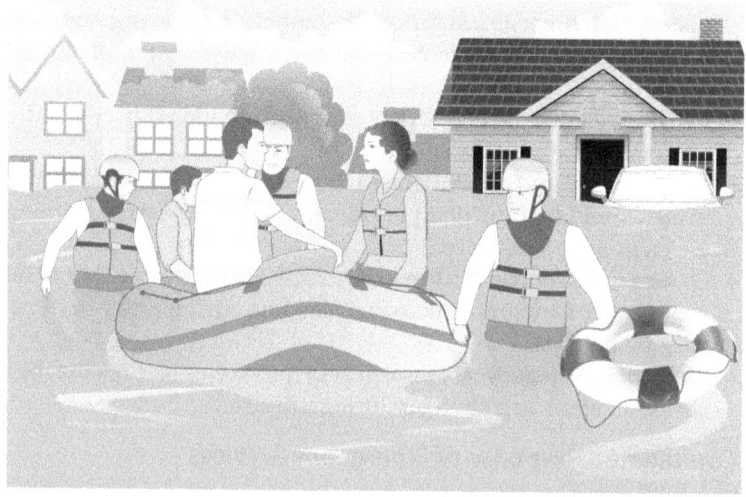

Fig. 12.1.3: Police personnel rescuing victims of floods.

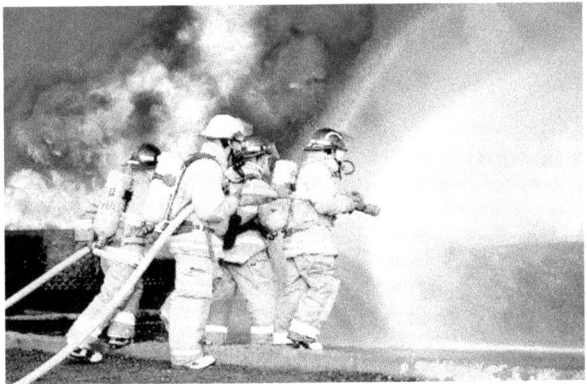

Fig. 12.1.4: Firemen at work to extinguish fire.

Ambulance Services

The ambulance services play an important role during disaster and emergency situations by:
- Deliver health services by responding during emergency situations.
- Manage pre-hospital emergencies healthcare services.
- Transport patient to the appropriate hospital and medical facilities.
- Ensure continuity of care.

Civil Defense Personnel

The role of civil defense personnel is to coordinate the activities of the police and firemen. The tasks usually performed are:
- Coordinating the services of the police and firemen.
- Organizing and directing.
- Set up communication system.

Armed Forces

The roles of the armed forces are (**Fig. 12.1.5**):
- Assist police and firemen in their functions as needed.
- Organize and establish the pattern of:
  - Communication.
  - Rescue.
  - Evacuation.
  - First aid.
  - Transportation of victim.
  - Direct relief operation.

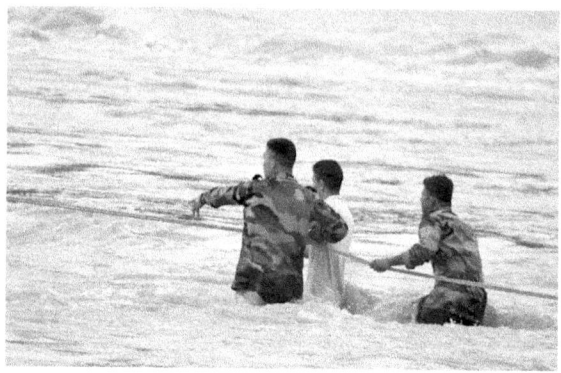

Fig. 12.1.5: Armed forces saving victims of floods.

Doctor

The primary role of the doctors is to save lives and to prevent further trauma and injury. The task responsibilities of doctors are:
- First aid
- Surgical support
- Evacuation decision
- Triage
- Provide basic life support measure to the victim in critical condition, i.e., basic airway maintenance and control of serious bleeding.

Nurses

- Nurses play an important role in disaster operation:
- Assessment of victim
- Triage
- Documentation of triage findings
- Regulating flow of victim for first aid
- First aid
- Evacuation
- Giving basic life support measures to the victims in critical condition, i.e., basic airway maintenance and control of serious bleeding.

Red Cross Personnel

The role of the Red Cross personnel is to render assistance care by:
- Ambulance services
- Setting up first aid team

- Providing food, drink, and temporary shelters for victims and rescuers.
- Supplying drugs and equipment.
- Helping in rehabilitation.
- Supply of clothes, blankets, etc.

Volunteers

Volunteers' role, during rescue operation, has been greatly realized. The genuine contribution of 'public spirited' citizens should provide the bulk of disaster operation in coordination with the professionally trained persons:
- Rescue
- First aid
- Evacuation.

Public Work Personnel

Public work personnel may perform any action, which lessen the chance of a secondary disaster. The tasks are:
- Removing roadblocks to clear traffic vehicles, dozers and ambulances.
- Prevention of any untoward effects, i.e., breakdown of power lines, water lines and gas lines.
- Assistance to firemen in obtaining adequate water for fire firefighting.
- Removing victims from under debris.

Disaster Management Agencies

Some of the National and International agencies for disaster management are mentioned below:

National Agencies

1. **National Disaster Management Plan (NDMP):** The National Disaster Management Plan was released in 2016. The aim of NDMP is to make India disaster resilient and significantly reduce the loss of lives and assets. NDMP is based on:
    - Understanding disaster risk.
    - Improving disaster risk governance.
    - Investing in disaster reduction (through structural and non-structural measures).

- Disaster preparedness, early warning and building back better in the aftermath of a disaster.
2. **National Disaster Management Authority (NDMA):** National Disaster Management Authority is the highest body for Disaster Management in India, headed by the Prime Minister of India. State Disaster Management Authorities (SDMAs) headed by respective Chief Ministers of the States function under NDMA. Members of the NDMA includes:

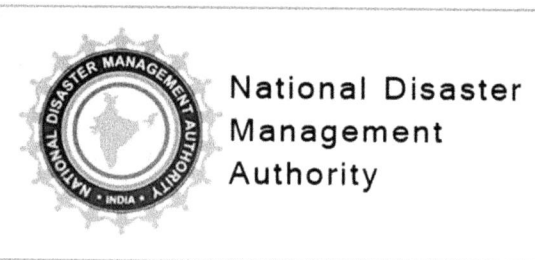

Chairman: Prime Minister of India.

Vice chairman: Cabinet Minister.

Members: 8 members with the status of ministers of state.

Objectives of NDMA: To lay down policies, plans and guidelines to ensure timely and effective response to disasters.

Responsibilities of NDMA includes:
- Develop policies on disaster management.
- Give approval for national plans as well as plan prepared by the Ministries or departments of the Government of India.
- Lay down guidelines to be followed by state authorities and different ministries or departments of the government of India.
- Enforce and implement the planned policies and guidelines.
- Propose funds for the purpose of mitigation.
- Provide support to disaster affected countries.
- Take up certain new measured for the prevention of disaster.
3. **National Disaster Response Force (NDRF):** The National Disaster Response Force was established under section 45 of Disaster management Act, 2005. The main objective of this agency is to provide specialized response to natural and man-made disaster. Natural Disaster Reference Database (NDRD) has to function under the general superintendence, direction and control of the National Disaster Management Authority (NDMA) and under command

and supervision of Director General, NDRF. The main function of NDRF includes:

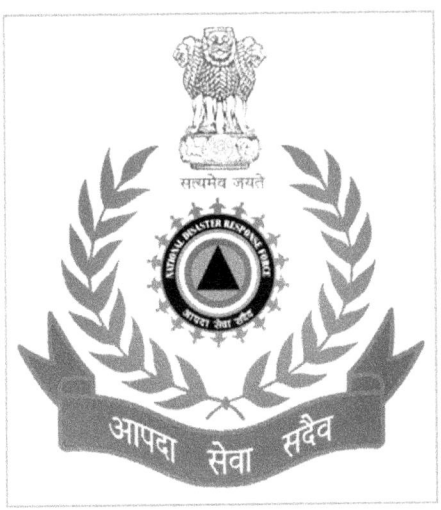

- Provide multi-disciplinary, multi-skilled, high-tech force capable of dealing with all kinds of disasters.
- Services are provided by highly trained personnel's from BSF, CRPF, CISF and ITBP.

4. **National Institute of Disaster Management (NIDM):** National Institute of Disaster Management was formulated under an Act of Parliament. The vision is to develop a premier institute for capacity development in India and the region.

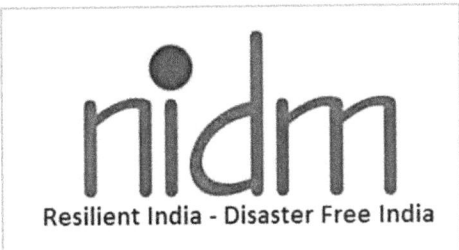

- Under disaster management Act 2005, NIDM is responsible for human resource development, capacity building, training, research, documentation and policy advocacy in the field of disaster management.

- NIDM also contributed by providing technical support to the state Government by linking with disaster management centers (DMCs) in the administrative training institutes (ATIs) of the States and Union Territories.
- The national focal point and host organization for the SAARC Disaster Management Centre (SDMC) is NIDM.
5. **National Executive Committee (NEC):** The chairperson for NEC is the Union Home Secretary. The members of NEC includes Secretaries to the Government of India. NEC works by preparing National Plan for Disaster Management as per the National Policy on Disaster Management.
6. **State Disaster Management Authority (SDMA):** SDMA is supervised by Chief Minister of the respective state. The work of SDMA on disaster management is assisted by State Executive Committee (SEC). Some of the responsibilities of SDMA includes:
   - Develop awareness campaign in the state.
   - Risk and vulnerability assessment for occurrence of disaster.
   - Preparation of disaster management policies.
   - Preparation of mitigation plans.
   - Ensure that mock drills for disaster response are being conducted.
   - Development of recovery framework for the state.
   - Lay down, review and update state level response plans and guidelines.
7. **District Disaster Management Authority (DDMA):** The head of District Disaster Management Authority is the District collector, Deputy Commissioner or District Magistrate depending on the situation. The co-chairperson is the elected representatives of the local authority. The work of DDMA is to ensure that the guidelines framed by the NDMA and the SDMA are followed by all departments of the district levels.
8. **Local authorities:** Municipalities, District and Cantonment 11 Institutional and Legal Arrangements Boards, Town Planning Authorities, and Panchayati Raj Institutions (PRI), which oversee and manage civic services, are examples of local authorities that work towards disaster management.

International Agencies

1. **International strategy for disaster reduction (ISDR):** ISDR was established in December 1999. ISDR is led by the United Nations

(UN) special representative of the Secretary-General for Disaster Risk Reduction (SRSG). The headquarters is located in Geneva, Switzerland with over 100 staff. The work of ISDR includes:

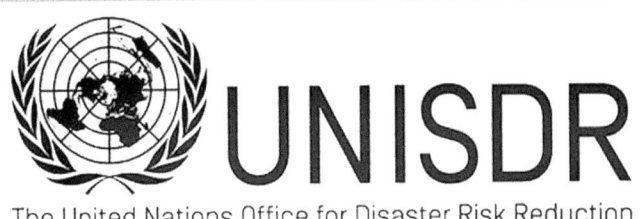

The United Nations Office for Disaster Risk Reduction

- Ensure disaster risk reduction (DRR) by applying it to climate change adaptation.
- Increasing the investment for disaster risk reduction (DRR).
- Building disaster resilient cities, schools and hospitals.
- Strengthening the international system for DRR.
- Implementation of Sendai.

2. **The United Nation and its organization:**
   a. **United Nations Disaster Management Team (UNDMT):** UNDMT is chaired by the UN resident co-ordinator. The United Nations Development Program (UNDP) disaster focal point officer serves as secretary for the UNDMT. The responsibilities of UNDMT includes:
      - Ensure effective emergency response.
      - Provide assistance to the government of the disaster effected countries for rehabilitation, reconstruction, and disaster mitigation.
      - Co-ordinate all disaster related activities provided by the United Nations.
      - Assist United Nations in avoiding wastes, duplications or competition for resources by UN agencies.
      - Co-ordinate with the emergency management team of the disaster affected countries.
   b. **United Nations Office for the Co-ordination of Humanitarian Affairs (OCHA):** OCHA is part of the UN Secretariat and is headed by an Under-Secretary-General. Office of OCHA is situated in Geneva and New York. The work of OCHA includes:

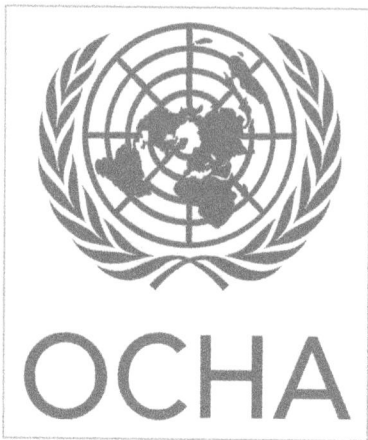

- Geneva office acts as the focal point for emergency operational support and relief co-ordination as well as for disaster mitigation.
- In New York, policy co-ordination, policy planning, early warning and response to complex emergencies are performed.
- OCHA works functions twenty-four-hour.
- Issuing information reports and situation reports.
- Involvement of teams in disaster affected area by co-ordinating relief efforts, launching joint UN appeals etc.
- In an emergency, OCHA has a Central Emergency Revolving Fund (CERF) that can be used to provide the UN Resident Co-ordinator with urgent funds, the funds can be reimbursed by the agency.

c. **United Nations Development Programme (UNDP):** UNDP works on disaster management by focusing on development aspects of the disaster. The work includes:

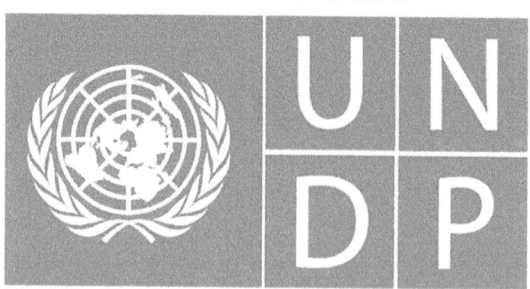

- Providing technical assistance to institution-building related to disaster management.
- Including long-term risk reduction and preparedness in standard development planning and programs.
- Assist in planning and implementation of rehabilitation and reconstruction of disaster effected area.
- Defining new development strategies that incorporate risk reduction measures relevant to the affected area.
- Evaluating the impact of large settlement of refugees and developing strategies to deal with it.
- Providing technical assistance to authorities managing major emergency operations of extended duration.

d. **United Nations High Commissioner for Refugees (UNHCR):** The aim of UNHCR response is to provide protection to persons of concern to the organization (Refugees) and ensure that the necessary assistance reaches them in time. Responsibilities of UNHCR includes:

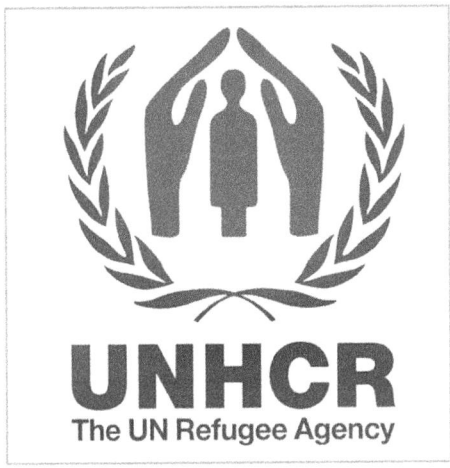

- Providing material assistance to survival refugees through adequate food, supplies, health care, shelter, water and sanitary facilities, clothing and essential community services.
- Provide financial assistance to refugees and displaced persons in emergency situations through UNHCR Emergency Fund.
- UNHCR has Emergency Preparedness and Response Section (EPRS) supervise by 5 officers.

e. **United Nations Children Fund (UNICEF):** In times of crisis (can be any crisis), UNICEF works to meet the immediate needs of children and mothers while taking into account the urgency of those needs and the resources at hand. Emergency response unit of UNICEF are situated in New York, Geneva and Nairobi. The activities of UNICEF includes:

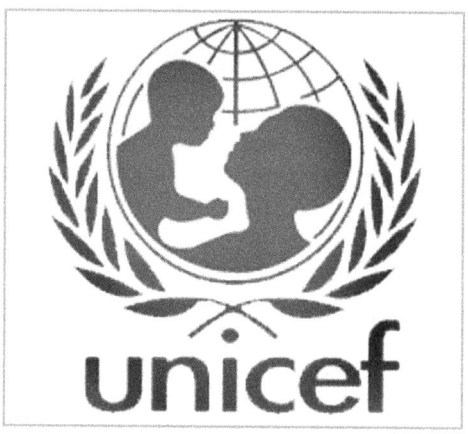

- Provides direct relief assistance in situations where immediate needs of children and mothers are not being adequately met.
- UNICEF concentrates on rehabilitation and long-term child survival and development objectives, in situations where the relief needs of mother and children can be met by the government.
- Provides special attention to the needs of children caught in conflict situations.
- UNICEF also focus on providing inputs in respect of health, social services, water and sanitation, with special attention to: the feeding and immunization of infants and young children: the restoration of safe water supplies and household food production.
- Conduct various initiatives to vulnerable communities and households to care adequately for their children, including increasing their earning opportunities (especially for women).
- Provide assistance to strengthen the management of emergency operations.

f. **World Food Programme (WFP):** WFP multilateral assistance accounts for approximately 25% of world emergency food aid. WFP provide services during emergency situations by:

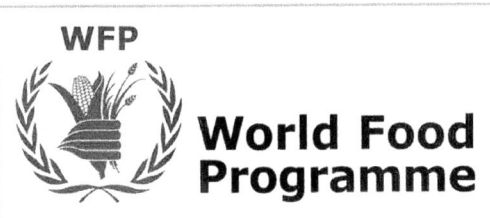

- Assist the government, other concerned agencies and local authorities in assessing requirements for emergency food aid, and in planning and managing food aid interventions.
- Depending on the resources at hand and the estimated demand for international food aid, UNICEF provide food aid to meet urgent food needs.
- Ensure coordination in the planning and delivery of food assistance from all sources, as well as any required logistical support and other supplementary inputs, and assist in mobilizing resources to do so.

3. **The Red Cross Movement:** The Red Cross Movement is composed of three elements:
   - *The National Red Cross or Red Crescent Societies:* The National Red Cross works by the principle of the Red Cross Services are provided by acting as auxiliaries to the public (governmental) authorities and services, and concentrate on activities concerned with public health-including first aid and primary health care and relief.
   - *The International Federation of the Red Cross and Red Crescent Societies (IFRCRCS):* The IFRC is a federation of the national societies world-wide. IFRCRCS headquarters are in Geneva, and its member societies are encouraged to engage in all kinds of humanitarian work to stop and lessen suffering in the world. When a disaster strikes, the IFRC can help the local society with needs assessments, resource mobilization, and relief activity planning. Personnel from other national societies may be requested and assigned under the federation's auspices, and IFRC delegates are frequently assigned to directly assist the national society.

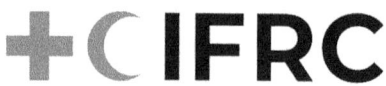

- *The International Committee of the Red Cross (ICRC):* The ICRC is the founder body of the Red Cross Movement. The International Committee of the Red Cross (ICRC) is a private, independent organization with its main offices in Geneva. It is also politically, ideologically, and religiously neutral. The ICRC offers shelter, medical attention, and material relief assistance to conflict victims. Additionally, ICRC organizes tracing services to locate and facilitate communication between estranged family members as well as visiting and tracing prisoners.

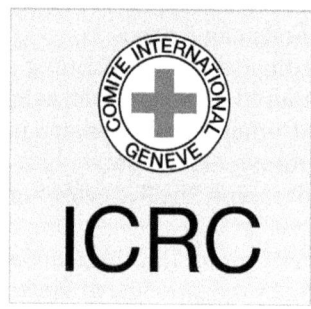

4. **World organization for animal health:** World organization for animal health works by:
    - Providing human and material resources that help in reducing the impact of disasters on animal health and welfare.
    - Building technical, management and good governance capacity of veterinary services.
    - Evaluating the performance of Veterinary services.

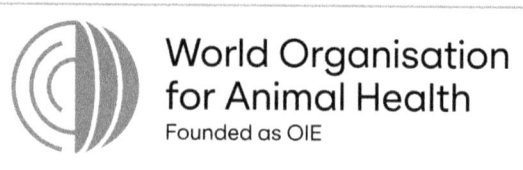

CHAPTER 12: Community Emergencies

- Collaborate with other organization such as FAO and WHO with regional organization to support veterinary authorities in developing surveillance, simulation models and other tools.
5. **Non-Governmental Organisations (NGO):** The Non-Governmental Organisations (NGO) working in emergency relief can be divided into two main categories, International NGO and local NGO. Some of the NGO includes:
   - Doctors without borders (MSF)
   - Direct relief international
   - Mennonite central committee
   - REACT international
   - City team international disaster response
   - Billy graham rapid response team
   - Hope worldwide
   - Plan India
   - CARE
   - World vision

REVIEW QUESTIONS

LONG ESSAYS

1. Define disasters. Explain the causes of disasters.
2. List the types of disasters and explain the effects of disasters.
3. Explain disaster triage and describe in details about victim assessment.

SHORT ESSAYS

1. Phases of disaster management.
2. Explain one national and internal agency involved in disaster management.
3. Explain all the coordinated response team of emergency services.
4. Principles of disaster management.
5. International guidelines for triage.

12.2: FIRST AID KIT

CHAPTER OUTLINE

- Contents for First Aid Kits
- Injuries and First Aid Supplies to be used

INTRODUCTION

A first aid kit is a collection of tools and supplies for administering first aid. It can be assembled for the purpose (by a person or an organization) or purchased fully assembled. The majority of first aid kits typically concentrate on treating trauma injuries, such as bleeding, bone fractures, burns, and infection control, and the vast majority of kits also contain bandages and dressings.

A first aid kit can be any size, color, or shape. Depending on the situation and the requirements of the manufacturer, the contents of the box may also change. National and international standards have guidelines that serve as a checklist for equipment and its use. The contents of first aid kits can vary greatly depending on the knowledge and experience of the person putting it together, the various first aid requirements of the location where it might be used, and changes in legislation or regulation in a particular area. Although many kits do not adhere to this standard, either because of how they are assembled or because they are not labelled with the ISO graphical symbol for first aid, it is the international standard for first aid kits.

CONTENTS OF FIRST AID KIT (FIG. 12.2.2)

Sl. No.	First aid kit	Use
1.	Torch: Battery powered.	
2.	Sterile hand gloves	Use on cuts, wounds, abrasions etc.
3.	Antiseptic liquid	Use on cuts, wounds, abrasions, bites
4.	Sterile water	To wash wound
5.	Crepe Bandage	Cover sprains and/or use on blunt injury of limbs/joints
6.	Triangular bandage	

Contd...

Contd...

Sl. No.	First aid kit	Use
7.	Tourniquet	To stop bleeding
8.	Compressed roller bandage	Use on wound with gauze or in making sling and tie splints
9.	Surgical cotton rolls	Cleaning e.g., clearing dirt, grime and debris with water/ antiseptic solution
10.	Adhesive plaster/ tape	To hold bandage in place
11.	Adhesive bandage	To use on cuts/wounds over body parts that may not require use of large bandages (if needed hair should be shaved to prevent discomfort or further injury)
12.	Sterile gauze	To cover cuts, wounds or abrasions for preventing infection
13.	Eye pads	Covering an injured
14.	Sterilized paraffin gauze	To use on burn or scald before covering it with any bandage
15.	Silver sulfadiazine ointment	Used on burns and scalds
16.	Mouth to mouth resuscitator	Used in assisting mouth to mouth breathing. An infection barrier for performing artificial respiration as part of CPR
17.	Scissor	For cutting bandage, cloth, tape etc
18.	ORS packets	Oral rehydration solution packets for dehydration
19.	Glucose powder	To be mixed with water as a drink for quick energy and/or rehydration
20.	Forceps	Can be used to hold sterile gauze or access areas that may not be easy to reach
21.	Safety pins	For holding bandages or clothes in place
22.	Splints	A strip of rigid material used for supporting and immobilizing a broken bone
23.	Additional supplies: • Ibuprofen • Hydrogen peroxide • Tweezers	 • Pain relief • Cleaning wounds • To remove splinters

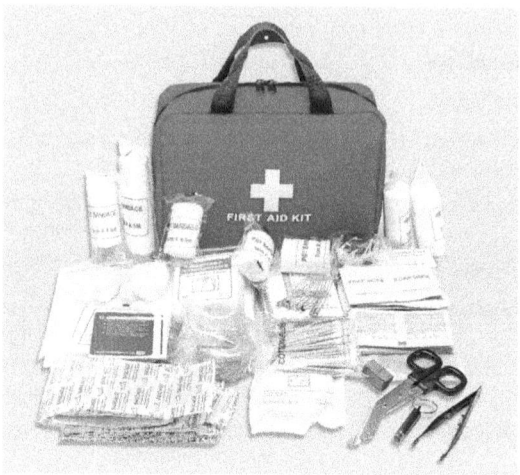

Fig. 12.2.2: First aid kit.

INJURIES AND FIRST AID SUPPLIES TO BE USED

1. **Gunshot wound:** Pressure bandages, compressed gauze tourniquets, and latex free gloves are used to control bleeding.
2. **Severed/crushed limb:** Tourniquet to stop hemorrhage/blood-loss.
3. **Deep wound:** Compressed gauze, abdominal dressing, compress bandage or blood stopping bandages.
4. **2nd and 3rd degree burns:** Sterile water, water-based gels saturated gauze and sterile gauze dressings.
5. **Broken Bone:** Triangular bandage, splinting material, elastic bandages and first aid tape.
6. **Cuts and scrapes**: Adhesive bandages, butterfly bandages, antiseptics, gauze pads, first aid tape, and gauze rolls.
7. **Minor burns**: Burn sprays and water-based burn gels are used to help relieve pain and treat the burn.
8. **Minor eye irritations**: Sterile eye irrigation solutions (eye wash) are used to rinse the eye from dust or dirt that may be irritating the eye.
9. **Sprains and strains:** Instant cold pack, elastic compression type products and splinting material like tongue depressors or an aluminum, moldable splint.
10. **Eye injuries:** Eye pads.

Index

Page numbers followed by *f* refer to figure and *t* refer to table.

A

Abdominal pain 135, 197
Abdominal thrusts 132
Abrasions 38, 39*f*
    signs of 38
Accident
    caused by 234
    history of 17
    transport 236
    victim, lifting of 126*f*
Acid 190
    burnt 177
    strong 207
Aconite poisoning 206
    symptoms 206
    treatment 206
Agricultural poisons 203
    treatment 204
Air passages, smaller 26
Airway 8
    opening 141
    patency of 9*f*
Airway obstruction 143
    assessment 142*f*
    causes 144
    first aid 145*f*
    first aid measures 144
        for partial 132
        for total 132
    foreign body 143
    general guidelines 144
    partial 131, 132
Alcohol poisoning 197
Alcoholic intoxication 189
Alkali 190
    burnt 177
    strong 207
Alveoli 26
Amanita phalloides 194, 195*f*

Ambulance
    loading head first in 127*f*
    loading stretcher in 126
    services 247
Ammonia 198
Amphetamines 196
Ancistrodon 213
Ankle
    bones 25
    dislocated 84*f*
    sprain 82*f*
Antirabic treatment 221
Apoplexy 155, 158
    signs 158
    symptoms 158
    treatment 158
Armed forces, roles of 247, 248*f*
Arms, examining 14
Arrhythmia, shock due to 69
Arsenic poisoning 190, 204
    symptoms 204
    treatment 205
Arteries 29
Arterioles 29
Asphyxia 128, 137, 155
    causes of 130
    signs of 194
    symptoms of 194
Aspirin 190, 207
    overdose 197
Asthma 136
    attack, causes of 136
    management of 137
    signs 136
    symptoms 136
Atropa belladonna 194, 195*f*
Avalanches 233
Back blow
    fail 145
    method 133*f*
Bandage 93
    ankle with triangular 102*f*

circular 95f
for back of chest 106
for chest 106
four-tailed 106, 109t
fractured
    arm 77f
    hip 107f
lower jaw 91f
purpose of 93
roller 99, 99t, 100f
shoulder 106
special 99, 106
tailed 106
triangular 77f, 101, 107f
types of 99
uses of triangular 102

B

Bandaging
    patterns used in 94
    principles of 94
    shifting patient after 108f
Barbiturate 196
    drugs 189
Basic life support 145
Bee sting 219
Belladonna 189
Bites 209
Black widow spider 211, 211f
    bite 213
Bleeding
    control 54
    first aid measures of 54
    internal 58
    moderate 242
    severe external 56
    special forms of 59
    varicose vein, direct pressure on 65f
Blizzard 235
Blood loss
    methods for controlling 55
    sustained 17
Blood pressure 244
Body parts, essential 20
Boils 51
Bones 22
    broken 262
    carpal 24
    cheek 23
    cranial 23f

displacement of 83
ethmoid 22
finger 25
frontal 22
functions of 22
hyoid 23
innominate 25
lacrimal 23
metacarpal 25
metatarsals 25
nasal 23
occipital 22
palatine 23
parietal 22
parts of 22
shin 25
sphenoid 22
tarsal 25
temporal 22
thigh 25
toe 25
types of 22
wrist 24
Boots, removing 18
Brain
    direct injury to 156
    traumatic injury to 86
Breathing 8, 9, 148
    check for 143
    difficulty in 86, 134, 135
    muscles of 27
Bronchioles 26
Bruise 45, 45f, 82, 83f
    signs 82
    symptoms 82
    treatment 83
Burn 171, 172
    assessment of 173
    classification of 172
    cold 172, 173f
    depth of 173
    first aid for 176f
    rope 173f
    severe 178, 242
    shock 69
    treatment of 175
    types of 172, 173f
    wound 174
        classification of 174t

Burns mouth and throat 179
 first aid measures 179
 signs 179
 symptoms 179
Bystanders 15

C

Calf muscle strain 81*f*
Capeline bandage 105, 105*f*
Capillary 29
 hemorrhage 54
Carbolic acid 190, 223
Carbon
 dioxide 198
 tetrachloride 198
Carbon monoxide 190, 207
 poisoning 199
  management 199
Cardiac tamponade, shock due to 70
Cardiopulmonary resuscitation 152*f*
 application of 147
 basic 128
 guidelines in 147
 steps in 146
Carotid pulse 143*f*
 checking 13*f*
Carrying chair 121, 123, 125*f*
Carrying sheet 121, 123, 125*f*
Case, management of 5
Casualty 15
Central nervous system 32, 188
Chair method 120, 120*f*
Chemical burns 172, 173*f*
Chemical burns in eye 181
 first aid measures 181
 signs 181
 symptoms 181
Chemical burns in skin 180
 first aid measures 180
 signs 180
 symptoms 180
 treatment 180
Chemical vapors 187
Chest
 thrusts 145
 tightness 134
 trusts method 133
 wounds, penetrating 47
Chest compression 8
 correct position for 150*f*
 with rescue breaths 150

Chin lift 9*f*
 to open airway 148*f*
Choking 129, 131
 causes 131
 management of 132
 signs 131
 symptoms 131
Cholera, epidemic of 235
Circulation 8
 check for 143, 143*f*
Circulatory system 20, 28
 blood vessels 29
 function 28
 heart 28
Civil defense personnel 247
Clavicle 24
 fracture of 76
Cleaning debris 235
Clothing, removing 17
Coat, removing 18
Cobra, common 214
Cold therapy 90
Collapsing buildings 9
Collar and cuff sling 109, 110*f*
Collar bone 24
Colubrines 215
Coma 156, 189
 diabetic 161
Community emergencies 232
Conchae, inferior 23
Concussion 86, 157, 157*f*
Cone-shaped shells 221
 first aid measures 221
Consciousness 154
 level of 85
 loss of 154
 state of 244
Contact with current, remove casualty
  from 184
Copper 200
Coral cuts 221
 first aid measures 221
Corrosive poisons 202
 first aid treatment for 190*t*, 203
Cradle method 115, 115*f*
Crash helmets, removing 18
Cresol 190
Cuts and scrapes 262
Cyanides 191

D

Datura poisoning 205
   symptoms 205
   treatment 205
Dead drunk 189
Deadly nightshade 194
Death cap fungus 194
Delirium, causing 189
Dental injury 91
Depressants 196
Diabetes 155
Diabetic coma
   signs of 161, 161*t*
   symptoms of 161
Diarrhea, causes of 201
Digestive system 20, 27
Direct pressure 55
Disaster
   causes of 234
   effects of 237, 237*f*
   management of 238
   man-made 234
   mitigation 241
   natural 233, 250
   phase of 238
   preparedness 239
   recovery 241
   rescuers, tips for 245
   response 240
   triage 241
   types of 233
   victim, care of 241
Disaster management 232, 239
   Act 251
   agencies 249
   phases of 239, 240*f*
   principles of 239
Disease, epidemics of 233
Disinfectants 190
Dislocation 73, 83
   signs 83
   symptoms 83
   treatment 83
Dispensaries 191
District Disaster Management Authority 252
Double T-bandage 106, 109*f*
Drag method 117, 117*f*
Dressings 93

Drowning 129, 137
   management 138
   prevention measures for 138
   signs 137
   symptoms 137
Drug
   causing hallucinations 197
   poisoning 196
Dry burns 172
Dry burns and scalds 177
   first aid measures 178
   signs 177
   symptoms 177

E

Ear
   bleeding from 62
   examine 13
   foreign body in 168
   pouring oil in 169*f*
Earthquakes 233, 235
Echis carinatus 213
Ejaculatory ducts 32
Elbow 106*f*
   bandage 105
   divergent spica of 98, 98*f*
   roller bandage for 100*f*
Electrical burns 172, 173*f*, 181
   first aid measures 183
   signs 183
   symptoms 183
Electrical contact 9
Electrical wire using stick, removing 184*f*
Electroplating oil 191
Emergency
   cardiovascular care 146
   concept of 7
   resuscitation 141
   services, response of 245
Endocrine system 20, 29, 30*f*
   functions 29
   glands of 29
Epidemic, control of 235
Epiglottis 26
Epilepsy 155, 158
   first aid for 159*f*
   major 158
   minor 158

treatment 159
types 158
Epistaxis 60
Excessive heat, effects of 155, 161
Excretory system 20, 31
Exhaust fumes 190
Explosion 236
Extinguish fire 247*f*
Extreme temperature 227
Extremity, injury to 89
Eye
   affected by snow blindness 185*f*
   cornea of 185
   examine 12
   foreign body in 167
   injuries 262
   irritations, minor 262
   removing foreign body from 168*f*
   wounds 43

F

Face 23
   burnt 176
   examine 12
Fainting 162
   prevention 162
      measure for 163*f*
   signs 162
   symptoms 162
   treatment 162
Feet elevation 71*f*
Female reproductive system 32
Femur 25
   fracture of 78
Fibula 25
Figure-of-eight 96, 97*f*
Fire 9, 236
Fireman's lift and carry 116, 117*f*
Firemen 246, 247*f*
First aid 3, 129*t*
   care 213
   diagnosis 4
   disposal 5
   golden rules of 6
   management 71
   measures 38, 40-47, 50, 57-59, 62-66, 78, 86, 87, 129
   outline of 3
   scope of 4
   treatment 5, 202, 203

First aid kit 260, 262*f*
   contents of 260
Fits 189
Five and five approach 133*f*
Flood 236
   acid burn area 176*f*
   victims of 248*f*
Fold bandage 101
Food poisoning 200
   signs 200
   symptoms of 200, 201*f*
Foot
   bandage 103
      triangular 104*f*
   bones of 25
Fore-and-aft carry method 119, 120*f*
Forearm, fracture of 78
Foreign body 166
Four-handed seat 118, 119*f*
Fracture 25, 73
   causes of 73
      brittle bones 73
      direct force 73
      diseased bone 73
      indirect force 73
      muscle action 73
   closed 74
   communicated 74
   complicated 74
   compound 25, 74
   depressed 74
   first aid treatment of 74
   green stick 74
   impacted 74
   multiple 242
   open 74
   pathological 25
   signs of 74
   simple 25, 74
   special cases of 75
   symptoms of 74
   types of 73, 74
Free nerve ending 33
Frostbite 225
   first aid measures 226
   signs 225
   stages of 226*f*
   symptoms 225
   treatment 226
Full face helmet, removing 19

G

Gas
  fume 9
  poisoning 189
    causes 188
    stoves 190

H

Hailstorms 233
Hallucinations 197
Hallucinogens 196, 197
Hand
  and fingers, joints of 26
  bandage 102
    triangular 103*f*
  bones of 25
  palm of 44
  placement for chest compression, proper technique of 150*f*
  seats 118
Hanging 129, 139
  signs 139
  symptoms 139
Head
  and neck, sides of casualty 88*f*
  examining 12
  severe pain in 85
Head injuries 85
  signs of 85, 86
  symptoms of 85, 86
Head tilt 9*f*
  chin raise 141
Headache 135
Heart attacks 155
  shock due to 70
Heat cramps 229
  first aid measures 229
  signs 229
  symptoms 229
Heat exhaustion 228
  first aid measures 229
  signs 229
  symptoms 229
Heat rash 229, 230*f*
  first aid measures 230
  signs 229
  symptoms 229
Heatstroke 227
  first aid measures 228

signs of 227, 228*f*
symptoms of 227, 228*f*
Heimlich maneuver 132, 132*f*
Hemorrhage 37, 53, 54
  accidental 53
  classification of 53, 54*fc*
  first aid measures of 54
  internal 54
  management of 56
  postpartum 54
  primary 53
  secondary 53
  signs of 54
  symptoms of 54
Heroin 196
Hip
  bandage 106
  bones 25
Hornet sting 219
Household poisons, first aid measures for 195
Human anatomy 21*f*
Human body system 20
Human crutch 115, 115*f*
Human life, loss of 233
Humerus 24
Hurricane 234
Hydrogen cyanide gas 198
Hypodermic syringe 188
Hysteria 155
Hysterical fits 160
  signs 160
  symptoms 160
  treatment 160

I

Illness, history of 17
Incised wound, signs of 40
Indian hemp poisoning 205
Industrial gases 187
Industrial poisons 198
  classification 198
Infantile convulsions 155, 160
  signs 160
  symptoms 160
  treatment 161
Ingestion 188
Inhalation 187
Injured persons, transport of 114

Index

Injury
- associate 17
- multiple 11
- physical 237

Innumerable disasters strike 232
Insect bite
- first aid management of 210
- severe reaction of 209

Insulin coma 161, 161*t*
- signs of 161*t*

Insulin overdose 155, 161
- signs of 161
- symptoms of 161

Integumentary system 21, 33
Iodine 207
Irritants 202
Ischemia, shock due to 70
Izal 190

J

Jacket, removing 18
Jellyfish sting 220
- first aid measures 220

Joint 25
- and muscles, first aid to 80
- bandage 103
  - triangular 104*f*
- synovial 26

K

Kerosene 207
Kidneys, organs associated with 31
King cobra (hamadryad) 214
Knee cap 25
Krait *(Bungarus)* 214

L

Laburnum anagyroides 194, 195*f*
Lacerated wound, signs of 41
Landslide 233
Large arm sling 79*f*, 102, 109, 110*f*
Larynx 26
Leg
- elevation 71*f*, 163*f*
- examining 14
- fracture, positioning for 80*f*

Life, loss of 237

Limb
- crushed 262
- pressure bandage on 86*f*
- severed 262

Lips, examine 12
Loaded stretcher
- lifting of 126
- lowering 126

Lock jaw 46
Locust 233
Log-roll technique 89, 90*f*
Lower jaw injury 91
Lower leg, fracture of 79
Lower limbs 25
Lysergic acid diethylamide 196
Lysol 190

M

Male reproductive system 32
- parts of 32

Mandible 23
Many-tailed bandage 107, 109*f*
Mask form, dressing shape in 176*f*
Mass casualty management 245
Maxilla 23
Meissner's corpuscle 33
Mennonite central committee 259
Mercury 191, 208
Metals 190
Minor burns 262
- and scalds 178

Miscarriage 66
Morphia 191
Morphine 208
Mouth 12
- bleeding from 63

Mouth-to-mouth respiration twice 146
Multiple casualties 11
Muscle injuries 73
Musculoskeletal injuries 73
Musculoskeletal system 20, 22
Myocardial tumor, shock due to 70

N

Narcotics 196
Narrowed airway 136*f*
National Disaster Management Authority 250

Index

National Disaster Management Plan 249
National Disaster Response Force 250
National Executive Committee 252
National Institute of Disaster Management 251
National Red Cross 257
Natural phenomena at earth's surface 233
Nature, violence of 233
Neil-Robertson stretcher 121, 124, 125f
Nerve poisons 203
    first aid treatment 203
Nervous system 21, 32
Nervous tissue 33
Neutralize 192
Nitrous fumes 198
Nose 26
    bleeding 60
        first aid for 61f
    examine 12
    foreign body in 169

O

Obstructed alveoli 136f
Open face helmet, removing 18
Opium 191

P

Pacinian corpuscle 33
Palm
    bandaging 77f
    roller bandaging for 100f
Paraffin petrol 191
Paralysis 244
Patella 25
    fracture of 80
Patient assessment 141
Pelvic girdle 25
Pelvis 25
    fracture of 78
Penis 32
Peripheral nervous system 32
Person's clothes catch fire 175
Phalanges 25
Pharynx 26
Phenol 223
Phosphorus 191

Photography 191
Physical examination 12
Pick-a-back 115, 116f
    reverse 116, 116f
Pit viper 213
Placenta, premature detachment of 54
Poison 187, 190, 191, 207, 208
    action and effects 188
    common 204
    entry into body, mode of 187
    household 193f
    infected 189
    ingested 188
    nature of 187
    sources of 206, 207t
    types of 187, 193
Poisoning 187
    bites and stings 187
    determination by first aider 189
    treatment of 191
Poisonous Colubrines land snakes 214t
Poisonous fish 188
Poisonous fume 9
Poisonous gas
    common 135
    management of suffocation by 135
    suffocation by 129, 135
Poisonous plants 194
Poisonous reptiles 188
Poisonous snakes 214f
Poisonous substance
    drinking 188
    eating 188
Poisonous vipers land snakes 213t
Portuguese man-of-war 220
    first aid measures 220
Postexposure prophylaxis, first aid measures of 223
Potassium permanganate 207
Povidone iodine 223
Prostate glands 32
Prussic acid 189, 191
Psychological trauma 237
Public work personnel 249
Pulmonary vascular obstruction, shock due to 70
Pulse 244
Punctured wounds, signs of 41
Pupils 244

R

Rabies 221
  immunoglobulin 223
  signs in
    dog 222
    human 222
  symptoms in
    dog 222
    human 222
  transmission of 221*f*
Radiation 185
  burns 172, 173*f*
Radius 24
Reassure casualty 6
Red Crescent Societies 257
Red Cross movement 257
Red Cross personnel 248
Reef knot 94
Reproductive system 20, 31
Rescue phase 238
Respiration 244
  artificial 9*f*, 184
  external 26
  internal 26
Respiratory emergencies 128, 129
Respiratory system 20, 26, 27*f*, 136*f*
  organs of 26
Resuscitation 145, 152
Ribs, fracture of 76
Road accidents 8
Roller bandage 99, 99*t*, 100*f*
  rules for application of 101
Rule of nines 174, 175
Russell's viper *(Daboia)* 213

S

Safety 8
Salmonella 200
  poisoning 201
Scalds 171, 172, 173*f*
  severe 178
  treatment of 175
Scalp bandage 105
  triangular 105*f*
Scalp wound 59
  direct pressure on 60*f*
Scalp, bleeding from 86
Scapula 24
Scene safety 141
Scoop stretcher 121, 123, 125*f*
Scorpion sting 219
  first aid measures 219
  signs 219
  symptoms 219
Scrotum 32
Sea urchin sting 220
  first aid measures 220
Sedatives 208
Seminal vesicles 32
Sensory organs 20, 30
  ear 30
  eye 30
  nasal cavity 30
  skin 31
  tongue 31
Sensory receptor 33
Shelter 6
Shirt, removing 18
Shock 10, 37, 68, 155
  anaphylactic 70, 155
  cardiogenic 69
  causes of 68
  circulatory 70
  classification of 69
  dehydration 69
  distributive 70
  hemorrhagic 69
  hypovolemic 69
  insulin 161
  neurogenic 70
  obstructive 70
  septic 70
  stages of 69
  surgical 69
  treat for 86
  types of
    circulatory 70
    distributive 70
Shoes, removing 18
Shoulder blade 24
Single first aider, method of
    transportation for 115
Sinusoids 29
Skeletal muscles 26
Skeleton, appendicular 24
Skin 167*f*
  anatomy of 33*f*
  functions of 34
  pale 70
  sensory receptors of 33

Skull 22
  anatomy of 23*f*
  fracture of 75
Slings 109
  bandage, application of 106*f*
  improvised 111
  types of 109
Smoke
  management of suffocation by 135
  suffocation by 129, 134
Smoke inhalation 137
  management 137
  signs 137
  symptoms 137
Snake 213
  examination of 218
  venom, effects of 215
Snake bite 218
  first aid measures for 216
  signs 215
  symptoms 215
  treatment 216
  tying piece of cloth above 217*f*
Sniffing 196
Snow blindness 185
Snowstorms 233
Socks, removing 18
Soft tissue injury 90
Solvent inhalation 196
Spermatic cords 32
Spider 210
  bite, general first aid measures for 212
  brown recluse 211, 212*f*
Spinal cord
  injuries 85, 87
  signs for damage 87
  symptoms for damage 87
Spinal injury 87
  patient, lifting of 76*f*
Spine
  examining 13
  fracture of 75
  injuries to 242
Spiral bandage
  reversed 94, 96*f*
  simple 95*f*
Splint 111, 113
  types of 112*f*
Splinter out, removing 167*f*
Splinters 166
  first aid measures 167
  signs 166
  symptoms 166
Sprain 81, 262
St John sling 111, 111*f*
Staphylococcal poisoning 200
State Disaster Management Authority 252
Sterilize tweezers 167*f*
Stimulants 196, 197
Stings 209
Stomach, foreign body in 170
Stop burns, using blanket to 176*f*
Strain 80, 262
Strangling 139
Stretcher 121, 126*f*
  closing 122
  opening 122
  paraguard 121, 124, 125*f*
  standard 121, 122, 125*f*
  testing 122
  transporting casualty to 124
  types of 122, 125*f*
  utila folding 121, 123, 125*f*
Stroke 164
  first aid measures 164
  signs 164
  symptoms 164
  treatment 165
Strychnine 189, 191, 208
Stump, recurrent bandage of 98, 99*f*
Suffocation 134
  causes 135
Sunburn 230
  first aid measures 231
  signs 230
  symptoms 230
Swallowed poisons 188, 189, 202
  treatment of 202
  type of 202
Switch off current 183

T

Talk with victims 245
T-bandage 106, 109*f*
Teeth 12
    examine 12
Temperature, effects of 225
Testes 32
Tetanus infection 46
Thermostat 225
Thoracic cage 24
Threat phase 238
Throat
    fishbone in 170
    foreign body in 170
Throttling 139
Thumb, spica of 97, 97*f*
Tibia 25
Tissues within throat, swelling of 129
Tornadoes 233, 235
Total airway obstruction 131, 132
Trachea 26
Tranquilizers 196
Transportation, methods of 114
Tremors 197
Triangular bandage 79*f*
    steps for application of 101
Trichloroethylene 198
Trolley bed 121, 123, 125*f*
Trousers, removing 18
Trunk, examining 13
Tsunamis 233
Two handed seat 118, 119*f*

U

Ulcer 50, 51*t*
    treatment for acute 51
    types of 51
Ulna 24
Ultraviolet light 185
Unconscious patient 10*f*, 147
    management of 155
Unconsciousness 9, 154, 156
    causing deep 189
    common causes of 155
    degree of 154
    early stage of 198
    later stage of 198
    treatment of 162
United Nations Children Fund 256
United Nations Development Programme 254
United Nations Disaster Management Team 253
United Nations High Commissioner for Refugees 255
Upper limb
    fractures of 76
    shoulder girdle with 24
Urethra 32

V

Vaginal bleeding 65
    symptoms 65
Varicose veins, bleeding in 64
Veins 29
Venules 29
Vertebral column 24
    movement of 24
Vest, removing 18
Victim
    assessment 141, 142*f*, 142*t*, 242
    design tasks for 245
    listen to 245
    transportation of 247
Violent windstorms 235
Viper 215
Vision difficulty 86, 134
Vital body parts 20
Volatile chemicals 198
Volcanic eruption 233
Volunteers 249
    role 249

W

Warfare, caused by 234
Wasp sting 219
Weather 6
Welder's flash 185
Wheelchair method 121

Windstorms 233
  cyclone 233
  hurricane 233
  typhoon 233
Wood splinters embedded 167*f*
Wound 37, 44
  abdominal 48
  deep 262
  gunshot 42, 43*f*, 262
  incised 39, 39*f*
  infected 46
  lacerated 40, 40*f*
  punctured 41, 41*f*
  scalp 59
  types of 38, 90
  with elevation, direct pressure of 56*f*
Wrist joint connecting forearm, roller bandaging for 100*f*

Z

Zygomatic bones 23

EU GSPR Authorised Reprsentative
Logos Europe, 9 rue Nicolas Poussin
1700, La Rochelle, France
Phone: +33 (0) 6 67 93 73 78
E-mail: contact@logoseurope.eu

www.ingramcontent.com/pod-product-compliance
Ingram Content Group UK Ltd.
Pitfield, Milton Keynes, MK11 3LW, UK
UKHW021832140426
5217IPUK00021B/1401